# Vitamania

**HEALTH AND MEDICINE
IN AMERICAN SOCIETY**

series editors
Judith Walzer Leavitt
Morris Vogel

# Vitamania
## *Vitamins in*
## *American Culture*

**RIMA D. APPLE**

**RUTGERS UNIVERSITY PRESS**
**New Brunswick, New Jersey**

Library of Congress Cataloging-in-Publication Data

Apple, Rima D. (Rima Dombrow), 1944–
    Vitamania : vitamins in American culture / by Rima D. Apple.
        p.      cm. — (Health and medicine in American society)
    Includes bibliographical references and index.
    ISBN 0-8135-2277-3 (cloth : alk. paper). — ISBN 0-8135-2278-1
(paper : alk. paper)
    1. Vitamins in human nutrition—Social aspects—United States.
I. Title.  II. Series.
QP771.A67    1996
615'.328—dc20                                                    95-43281
                                                                      CIP

British Cataloging-in-Publication information available

# Contents

List of Illustrations     vii

Acknowledgments     ix

**INTRODUCTION**
"Perhaps Your Diet Is Too Modern"
The Discovery of Avitaminosis     1

**CHAPTER 1**
"They Need It Now"
Popular Science and Advertising in the Interwar Period     13

**CHAPTER 2**
"To Protect the Interest of the Public"
Vitamins, Marketing, and Research     33

**CHAPTER 3**
"Superior Knowledge"
Pharmacists, Grocers, Physicians, and Linus Pauling     54

**CHAPTER 4**
Miles One-A-Day
The History of a Vitamin Dynasty     85

**CHAPTER 5**
Acnotabs
Scientific Evidence in the Marketplace     109

CHAPTER 6
"Millions of Consumers Are Being Misled"
The Food and Drug Administration and Consumer Protection    125

CHAPTER 7
"Preserve Our Health Freedom"
Science in Consumer Politics    144

CHAPTER 8
"Intensity" Makes the Difference
Vitamins in the Political Process    158

CONCLUSION
Vitamania?
Vitamins in Late Twentieth-Century United States    179

Notes    199

Index    233

# Illustrations

**Figure 1-1**  Kitchen Craft Waterless Cooker advertisement  15

**Figure 1-2**  Red Heart Dog Biscuit advertisement  16

**Figure 1-3**  Squibb's Cod-Liver Oil advertisement  21

**Figure 1-4**  Squibb's Cod-Liver Oil advertisement  23

**Figure 1-5**  Oscodal advertisement  24

**Figure 1-6**  Squibb Adex Tablets-10 D advertisement  28

**Figure 2-1**  Bottled Sunshine advertisement  39

**Figure 2-2**  Hygeia advertisement  43

**Figure 2-3**  Wisconsin Alumni Research Foundation
advertisement  45

**Figure 3-1**  "Vitamin Capsules in Strange Surroundings"  56

**Figure 3-2**  "Keep 'em coming!"  60

**Figure 3-3**  Whelan drugstore  64

**Figure 3-4**  "Vitamize" window display, Newark, N.J.  66

**Figure 3-5**  "You have the upper hand!"  71

**Figure 3-6**  "You're the expert"  72

**Figure 3-7**  "Stop that cold!" window display  76

**Figure 4-1**  Miles One-A-Day advertisement  94

**Figure 4-2**  "Year 'Round: One-A-Day Vitamins for Your
Whole Family"  96

**Figure 8-1**  "What do Dietary Supplements and Dinosaurs
Have in Common?"  175

# Acknowledgments

Many people have supported and encouraged this project. It is my great pleasure to publicly thank them for their faith and assistance over the years.

I will begin in a sense where the book began, with the sources. Suzanne White Junod, FDA historian, first made me aware of the wealth of material available in the Food and Drug Administration Archives. She instructed me in the intricacies of the archive's structure and provided a most comfortable work environment. Through the years she and her fellow FDA historian John Swann have been of immeasurable assistance. Celeste Aaron made me welcome at the Miles Laboratories Corporate Archives; I value her knowledge and her friendship. Betsy Hamilton made the Consumers Union Archives and her home available to me during my visit to Yonkers; I am grateful for both. James Liebig aided my research in the University of Wisconsin Archives. Else Arnold and John R. Pike helped me locate records in the files of the Wisconsin Alumni Research Foundation. Howard Shuman graciously agreed to be interviewed about his work in the office of Senator William Proxmire; his thoughts and analysis were appreciated. Discussions with Professor Aaron Ihde aided my understanding of Harry Steenbock.

David Sandmire was the most conscientious and capable research assistant. He spent six months finding matrial scattered through the libraries of the University of Wisconsin. The results of his diligent search of periodicals and newspapers, government hearings, and the Congressional Record have strengthened this study.

Funding for this study has come from the University of Wisconsin Graduate School, the National Institutes of Health (grant number 1 RO1 LM05279-01), and the National Science Foundation (award number DIR-8720456). I am indebted to them for their financial assistance. Any opinions, findings, and conclusions or recommendations expressed in this material are those of the author and do not necessarily reflect the views of the National Science Foundation.

Several of the following chapters have been published previously in different form. I wish to thank the following: IOP Publishing Limited for permission to reprint from "Science in the Marketplace: Acnotabs and the Food and Drug Administration," *Public Understanding of Science* 2 (1993): 59–70; the University of Chicago Press and the History of Science Society for permission to reprint from "Patenting University Research: Harry Steenbock and the Wisconsin Alumni Research Foundation," *Isis* 80 (1989): 374–394; and Bowling Green State University Popular Press for permission to reprint from " 'They Need It Now': Advertising and Vitamins, 1925–1940," *Journal of Popular Culture* 22, 3 (1988): 65–83. Material from the Miles Laboratories Corporate Archives and the Consumers Union Archives are reprinted with permission of those organizations.

Colleagues have been generous with their time. James Harvey Young always provided wise counsel. Janet Joy, Robert Joy, Suzanne White Junod, Susan Lederer, Naomi Rogers, and John Warner never turned a deaf ear to another discussion of vitamins. I wish to thank Janet Golden, Suzanne White Junod, and Gregory Higby for their insightful and instructive comments on early drafts. At Rutgers University Press, Karen Reeds is an energetic, creative, and thoughtful editor.

Two other people deserve special thanks. Michael Apple has endured endless conversations about vitamins. His support and his confidence have been unwavering. He has kept me "on task." Diane Mary Chase Worzala has been a part of this project from the beginning, reading every chapter, every word, more than once. In gratitude and in friendship, I dedicate this book to her.

• • • • • • • • • • • • • • • • • • • • • • • •

# Vitamania

# INTRODUCTION

• • • • • • • • • • • • • • • • • • • • • • • • • • •

# "Perhaps Your Diet Is Too Modern"
## The Discovery of Avitaminosis

While more expensive than such things as gin rummy or Chinese crackers, vitamin-taking is every bit as popular, maybe more popular. . . . Helping to give the vitamin pills their great popular appeal, of course, is the fact that they come in small and highly scientific looking bottles. —Robert M. Yoder, "Vitamania," *Hygeia,* April 1942, pp. 264–265.

Health, profit, power—Americans have sought all three in vitamins.

Manufacturers spend millions of dollars promoting the benefits of their products; consumers spend billions of dollars buying hundreds of different vitamin pills. Vitamin capsules are "magic pills." We take vitamins if we are under stress or tired. Vitamins promise sexual potency; they cure colds. Many take vitamin pills "just in case." Athletes take vitamin pills to maximize their achievements. We tell our children to "eat your vitamins." We buy vitamin-enriched beauty soaps and skin lotions. Vitamins are sold as candy.

The billion-dollar vitamin industry thrives. It thrives in spite of the heated scientific controversy that rages over the value of vitamin pills. It thrives perhaps because of the controversy. Clearly vitamins are essential nutrients; people fall seriously ill when vitamins are missing from their diets. But do well-fed, middle-class Americans need to take vitamins?

The aim of this book is not to settle *that* question, but rather to explore why we buy vitamins. In the face of fierce disagreement among scientists about the answer, why has the American consumer's love affair with vitamins continued unabated for nearly a century?

● ● ● ● ● ● ● ● ● ● ● ● ● ● ● ● ● ● ● ● ● ● ● ● ● ● ● ● ● ● ● ● ● ● ● ●

The critical importance of trace nutrients to animals and humans was first demonstrated in the beginning of the twentieth century. Scientists identified beriberi, scurvy, and pellagra (along with a number of other less well known illnesses) as diseases caused by the lack of some mysterious components in the diet— diseases dramatically cured by simple changes in diet. Intensive biochemical research isolated one vitamin after another and then devised methods for synthesizing them and mass producing them cheaply.

The discovery of vitamins was a triumph of science. It demonstrated the power of science to disclose the secrets of nature and to use that knowledge in the service of humanity. Vitamins represented the hope of better things to come. Not surprisingly, American vitamin manufacturers appealed to science in their promotional campaigns for their products. Advertisement after advertisement told of the value of vitamins, a value proven scientifically. They insisted that true health could be achieved only with the aid of vitamin pills.

Consumers quickly learned that there was more to the science of vitamins than advertisements admitted. Among scientists the need for vitamin supplements was hotly debated. Some cavalierly dismissed the idea, believing we get all the vitamins we need from our daily diets. Others promoted daily vitamins, even megadoses.

Do vitamins protect against cataracts, or against cancer? How effective are large doses of vitamin C in warding off the common cold? Should we take vitamin E to reduce the risk of angina and heart attacks? Even more controversial, are there subclinical vitamin deficiencies we have yet to identify? Is there any connection between vitamins and optimal health? As some experts say yes and others just as confidently say no, the debate quickly moves beyond the narrow confines of the scientific arena. With health, wealth, and power at stake, more players enter the battle: other scientists, manufacturers, pharmacists, physicians, policy makers, politicians, vitamin retailers, and consumers themselves. This book takes note of all of them. It looks at pharmaceutical companies, large and small. It examines scientists and the effect of commercial considerations on research agendas. It studies experts in health and how the debates over vitamins shaped their professional identities and prestige. It investigates the motives of government officials who tried to limit the vitamin industry. It explores how politicians use this issue that stirs up so much passion. Above all, it listens to the voices of consumers who keep on taking their vitamins, no matter how much scientists fight.

Decade after decade, as we shall see, the same scenario is repeated: scientists report on the beneficial effects of vitamins; the media and particularly manufacturers publicize the claims; skeptical scientists declare that the American consumer is being hoodwinked; government agencies propose regulations to control the advertising, labeling, and sale of vitamin pills; and concerned consumers assert their right to take their vitamins without government interference.

This tale of vitamins in American culture underscores the ambiguous authority of science.[1] Science has often been regarded as a secular religion in modern America; we take its pronouncements as akin to gospel. Each participant in this controversy exploited this view of science. From one perspective, faithful vitamin takers have been brainwashed by vitamin companies who continue to hammer home their science of vitamins. Yet this book shows us that the American consumer rejects such a dogmatic view of science. It is significant that when scientists rancorously disagree, many Americans remain passionately committed to vitamins and to science. Scientific experts and expertise are not rejected unilaterally. It is only that consumers demand the right to decide for themselves, once a day, every day.

The power and hope of vitamins thrilled the American public, even before scientists had figured out the chemical structures and physiological actions of vitamins. The earliest notes about vitamins in the popular press, dating from the 1910s, stressed the miraculous cures possible with the knowledge of vitamins. Article after article emphasized the importance of vitamins for good nutrition to insure a healthy body, and each admitted that "they are still somewhat of a mystery to even the most learned scientist. They cannot be isolated and dissected, but they have been subjected to such study that we know where they are found, what they do, and why we must eat foods containing them."[2] By 1921 scientists recognized three vitamins: fat soluble vitamine A, water soluble vitamine B and water soluble vitamine C.[3] By 1940 the list had grown to over twenty.[4]

Yet while describing vitamins as miracles, writers invariably sounded a note of caution. Articles with titles such as "How One May Feast and Starve" warned that vitamins were related to the quality of food, not the quantity.[5] Authors described modern methods of food processing that could strip out these vital elements. So too could home cooking. Consequently, the American diet was found lacking in many nutrients. One estimate in 1925 determined that 87 percent of the people in this country were choosing the wrong things to eat.[6]

By the 1920s and 1930s, general interest and women's magazines were instructing their readers in many details of the science of vitamins. In a telling piece, Ruth F. Wadsworth, M.D., described the known vitamin deficiencies. Without sufficient vitamin C, the result was scurvy; without B, beriberi; without D, rickets; and without A, an eye condition "caused by a lack of function in the tear-producing glands." But these were only the most extreme conditions that could arise from vitamin deficiencies.[7] She and other authors downplayed the significance of gross vitamin deficiency diseases such as scurvy and rickets. Instead, readers were warned about subclinical deficiencies: "If we get enough of it to prevent the specific eye trouble, but still not enough, we have lowered resistance to disease of various kinds, intestinal disturbance and, in the young, a failure to grow." Not enough of vitamin B, for example, could result in nervousness and a lack of pep. Despite all these difficulties, Wadsworth concluded on a reassuring note: "All we need to do is to make sure that our diet is so balanced and so varied that we will get some of each one of the four important vitamins each day; we ought then to have some assurance that our general health will be better than it might be."[8] Wadsworth's advice is typical of the era: an explanation of the problems that could arise from a lack of vitamins and then the reassurance that the solution was a balanced diet.

That counsel slowly changed, however. As researchers developed methods for isolating and synthesizing vitamins, suggestions to incorporate the micronutrients into the American food supply multiplied as well. For example, take vitamin B. Though we now recognize a combination of micronutrients that are grouped together as the vitamin B complex, in the 1930s vitamin B was considered a single entity with an amazing range of functions. First and foremost, vitamin B was necessary to prevent beriberi,[9] but there was little danger of beriberi in this country, most authors agreed. Writers were concerned, however, that insufficient vitamin B had an adverse effect on appetite and digestion.[10] Thus, when vitamin B was isolated and then synthesized in the late 1930s, researchers proclaimed the health benefits of fortifying food with this important micronutrient. Dr. Norman Hayhurst Jolliffe, a psychiatrist in New York City, studied one thousand cases of alcoholism at Bellevue Hospital, identifying 22.6 percent with polyneuritis, a painful "widespread inflammation of the nerves," likened to beriberi. He successfully treated this condition with vitamin B. Others had considered polyneuritis in alcoholics to be caused by the alcohol itself, but Jolliffe concluded it was a function of vitamin B deficiency. Part of his evidence came from a bartender who drank fifteen ounces of whiskey every day for forty years with no indication of nerve damage. He would pour the one and a half ounces of whiskey into a ten-ounce bar glass and fill the remainder of the glass with milk. Jolliffe believed that the milk provided sufficient vitamin B. The doctor suggested that manufacturers might include a trace of the vitamin in their products or that consumers might add their own vitamin B.[11]

The availability of vitamin concentrates made such proposals feasible. One enterprising manufacturer produced V. V. Vitawater, promoted with the slogan, "Science says drink the new way." This sparkling tonic water contained "the necessary Vitamin B factor," explained one advertisement, "that helps to make you feel better." In a further acknowledgment of the power of science, the copywriter added that Vitawater "has been tested and approved by scientific authorities."[12]

Advice reiterated throughout the many vitamin articles pub-

lished in the first half of the century stressed the need for vitamins in the daily diet and warned that vitamins were fragile. Modern food processing could strip vitamins from food. Heating and
chopping could destroy the vitamin content of even the best food.[13]
Advertisers were well aware of the widespread concern that vitamin content might be compromised by the conditions of modern
life. One vitamin manufacturer pointedly warned, "Perhaps your
diet is too modern." Mirroring the worries discussed in numerous
articles in the popular press and reminding readers that "modern
processing may unavoidably rob certain important foods" of their
vitamins, an advertisement recommended the pharmaceutical
product Vitroetts as a "convenient economical source" of these
micronutrients.[14]

Advertisers did not invent this concern about America's nutrition. By the late 1930s, several studies documented the nation's
poor diet.[15] Contrasting the United States with the famine faced
by war-torn Europe, writers claimed that the American population
was starved for vitamins. Nutritionists and physicians proposed
three reasons for this lamentable state of affairs. First, people did
not eat enough vitamin-rich foods. Second, what they did eat had
lost much of its vitamin content through modern processing.[16]
The third reason was the Great Depression: many families did not
have enough money to purchase an adequate diet. Even more,
sufficient income did not insure appropriate nutrition; supposedly well-off middle-class Americans were not safe because
people were frequently ignorant about wholesome food and careless in their buying habits. As a result, "in all probability the nutritional diseases constitute our greatest medical and public health
problem," one physician determined, "not from the point of view
of deaths, but from the point of view of disability and economic
loss."[17] Others claimed that 40 percent of the American population suffered from inadequate nutrition. Admitting that specific
or acute avitaminosis, such as scurvy, beriberi, or rickets, was rare,
writers would describe "the millions of sub-clinical cases—persons
who are not sufficiently ill to require medical aid, yet who are
really not well."[18] Though commentators usually mentioned the

need to educate consumers about the latest discoveries in nutritional science and to teach them how to incorporate this information into their dietary plans, just as frequently writers complained about "impoverished food." Food available in stores had been depleted by milling practices, by the needs of long-distance transport (that necessitated the shipment of unripe fruit which lacked the vitamin content of fully mature fruit), and by large-scale distribution procedures (that employed long-term cold storage during which further vitamins were lost through oxidation).

One health-promoting alternative to denatured food was to enrich common foods with vitamins. During the Great Depression, under the direction of Harry Steenbock and the Wisconsin Alumni Research Foundation, many products were enhanced with the addition of vitamin D.[19] Another popular plan was the enrichment of flour. Groups such as the U.S. Department of Agriculture would have preferred to educate the public about wholesome food selection and food preparation, but they recognized that education was a long-term project. In the short term, especially since "too many young men were found unfit for military service in part because of poor nutrition," the agency wholeheartedly pushed for the enrichment of flour and the marketing of enriched white bread.[20] By 1946, manufacturers commonly added vitamins to flour, bread and rolls, cornmeal and grits, macaroni and spaghetti, breakfast cereals, oleomargarine, and milk.

In sum, the popular press was filled with articles in which science could give concern and hope to the American consumer. These publications often charged that the U.S. population suffered chronic famine. The American food supply was declining in quality. Improper storing and cooking could further decrease the vitamin content of the food on your table. But you could get sufficient vitamins in your diet if you were careful: careful about what you bought—preferably fresh fruits and vegetables, enriched flour, and enriched milk—and careful about how you served your fruits and vegetables—preferably raw or lightly cooked. And, to be on the safe side, you might add a tablespoon of wheat germ to your diet each day. Children certainly should have cod-liver oil.

These "additions" implied that the average middle-class American diet was not nutritionally sufficient. Quickly the pharmaceutical industry rushed in to fill the need.

Even before vitamins were isolated or could be synthesized, alert entrepreneurs built a vitamin industry on the promises of vitamin research. One of the first products was cod-liver oil, which will be discussed in the next chapter. But evolving research spurred manufacturers in other areas also. As early as 1925, one enterprising researcher suggested a procedure for producing vitamin tablets. "Orange peelings ground in a meat chopper, dried and ground in a coffee mill may be made into tablets by the addition of dehydrated orange juice acting as a binder." This method, its creator felt, would be particularly useful for those who did "not relish certain vitamine-containing vegetable products," such as spinach. With this tablet, you could attain the vitamins necessary for health and "avoid the censorship of the palate."[21] It is not clear whether any company chose to use this process, but just two years later there were at least twenty brands of commercial vitamin products advertised for their vitamin B content alone.[22]

The American Medical Association was most critical of the emerging industry. In articles and in editorials, starting as early as 1922, the organization called the commercial hype surrounding vitamins "a gigantic fraud."[23] Over and over again, the AMA campaigned against vitamin supplements, insisting that a diet lacking vitamins would give rise to gross vitamin-deficiency diseases. These conditions were the concern of the doctor. Otherwise, the solution lay in diet, not commercial vitamin pills.[24] Positioning themselves as the experts on vitamins and as the protectors of the public health, physicians frequently reminded the "befuddled consumer" to "get his vitamins from the garden and orchard rather than from the drug counter." According to AMA articles, vitamin pills were within the purview of the physician, not the layperson. Clearly, commercial vitamin pills undercut the authority of the medical practitioners to direct the patient's health.

Others were more willing to entertain the possibility that vitamin concentrates could be worthwhile. In *Ladies' Home Journal*, a senior chemist in the U.S. Department of Agriculture, Sybil L. Smith, counseled that vitamin B concentrates could be very helpful for nursing mothers.[25] Dr. Walter H. Eddy, director of the Good Housekeeping Bureau, referred to scientific studies conducted in university laboratories and the laboratories of *Good Housekeeping* to support his contention that vitamins A and D could enter the body through the skin. Citing this scientific and medical authority, he recommended skin creams and soaps manufactured with the addition of sufficient vitamins "to produce their health-giving benefits."[26] Indicative of the contradictory information presented in the popular press, just a few months earlier, *Hygeia* (the AMA's popular health magazine) had dismissed the idea that soaps could provide the body with necessary vitamins.[27]

Authors could recommend vitamin products because more vitamins were out on the market. Declining production costs helped fuel this expansion. Throughout the 1920s and 1930s, researchers assiduously investigating vitamins had isolated and even synthesized many of these micronutrients, laying the foundation for a lucrative industry.[28] These developments made vitamin concentrates easily available and significantly less costly. For instance, Vitamin $B_1$, extracted from rice polishings, once cost $300 a gram; by 1943 the price had dropped to 37 cents a gram. Costs of other vitamins declined similarly.

Another important impetus to the industry and the popularity of vitamin pills among middle-class Americans was World War II. Following the United States's entry into the war, stories continued to appear in the press about the deteriorating American food supply. Moreover, the pressure of the war placed a premium on an efficient workforce. Since the early 1930s, researchers had been studying the possible connection between vitamin intake and increased productivity. One such test concluded that workers regularly given cod-liver oil developed fewer colds and had less absenteeism than a control group.[29] At another factory, workers received vitamins as the result of a more personal experience. Leighton Wilkie, president of Continental Machines, believed

• • • • • • • • • • • • • • • • • • • • • • • • • • • • • • • • • •

that his greater resistance to colds resulted from daily doses of cod-liver oil and other vitamins. Consequently, he distributed vitamin capsules to his employees during the winter months.[30]

Such stories, coupled with patriotic fervor, inspired researchers to study more closely the relationship between vitamins and worker efficiency. If vitamins resulted in less fatigue, less inefficiency, and less illness, then they would improve productivity and thus help save lives and shorten the war. Various tests demonstrated just that. Time after time, researchers discovered that workers receiving vitamins had significantly lower rates of absenteeism, stayed in their jobs longer, and even scored higher on their merit ratings.[31] In another boost for the vitamin industry, factory workers' extensive use of vitamin pills convinced their friends and families to buy the products for home use.[32]

Supplementation was also proposed to foster positive labor relations. Dr. Russell N. Wilder of the Mayo Clinic demonstrated the power of thiamine, $B_1$, the anti-beriberi vitamin. He studied a group of female volunteers who were "sociable, contented workers." They were fed an "acceptable, palatable diet," but one without thiamine. In a few weeks, Wilder reported, their personalities had changed drastically; they quarrelled, became depressed, and tired easily: "They even went on strikes." Once thiamine was returned to their diets, it took only two days for them to become "their old selves again."[33] Claims such as these about vitamin $B_1$ were played for comic effect in Hollywood. A staid society husband in *The Gang's All Here* (1943) chides his wife for flirting with another man. The woman defends herself: "Can I help it if I am irresistible?" He corrects her: "It's that vitamin $B_1$. I told you you were taking too much. You're overdoing it." Hollywood's causal, farcical reference demonstrates that middle-class audiences were familiar with the effect of vitamin B on the psyche.

Rationing also aided the popularity of vitamin supplementation during the war. Rationing made it more difficult to obtain the foods necessary for a healthy, well-balanced diet, as vitamin manufacturers reminded consumers. No need to worry, though; Abbott Laboratories proudly announced the scientific justification for its "Victory" vitamins, which supplied the average adult's requirements of the six vitamins "now considered as all important for the maintenance of an adequate state of nutrition."[34]

Still, not everyone was convinced about the need for vitamin supplementation. One doctor, in 1942, was aghast at the "hundreds of thousands of dollars worth of vitamin concentrates" swallowed by the American public. He was sure that vitamins had become the "sport of quacks and the rich bonanza of the nostrum vendors." He and other commentators were adamant that one could and should get vitamins from one's daily diet.[35] Such debunkers joyfully pointed to each report that undercut the claims of vitamin advocates and then shook their heads in dismay as Americans continued to gulp down vitamins. Nevertheless, despite many articles in the popular press deriding the use of vitamin pills, the industry grew. Vitamin sales increased steadily through the 1930s, from slightly over $12 million in 1931 to more than $82.7 million in 1939. By 1942 total vitamin sales in this country had grown to over $130.8 million.[36] As later chapters document, statistics from the second half of the century show that many American consumers continue to buy nutritional supplements.

The development and use of vitamins intersect with many aspects of our society—economic, social, political, and even military. But, above all, the history of vitamins illustrates the many ways science is used to affect our lives. Pharmaceutical companies used science relentlessly in their promotions. At the same time, the popular press regularly publicized the latest scientific pronouncements and the miracles of vitamin therapy. Some writers did insist that vitamin pills were a waste of money better spent on healthful food; but even in their damning articles, the public learned more about the science of vitamins. Other champions included researchers, physicians, and government officials who aired their concerns about vitamins in the public media. Pharmacists too positioned themselves as consumer advocates and educators in the area of vitamin supplementation. Government actions, specifically attempts by the Food and Drug Administration to regulate the vitamin industry, focused the debate on the limits of regulation. Contradictory scientific claims and challenges to scientific authority abounded as scientists, physicians, manufacturers, retailers, and, most significantly, consumers argued about the need for vitamins. The dispute over government regulation gave consumers the opportunity to explain their faith in vitamins, based on their view of science.

In all this, the lack of scientific consensus was manifest; the confusion, conspicuous. Yet promoters and debunkers were united on one significant point: the answer to the question of vitamins would be found in science.[37] When scientists disagree, Americans do not stop believing in science; they just decide the matter for themselves. The controversy over vitamins provides a window for studying the authority of science in our society. For understanding the role of vitamins in American consumer culture, science is the crucible.

# CHAPTER 1

● ● ● ● ● ● ● ● ● ● ● ● ● ● ● ● ● ● ● ● ● ● ● ● ● ●

# "They Need It Now"

## Popular Science and Advertising in the Interwar Period

> Take some standard food, milk for instance, reduce it to its elements, extract all these elements—and you still have left "vitamines," without which life cannot endure. What are vitamines?—just that; that something that is left after everything has been removed. At least, so it seems to the layman.
>
> In a sense, vitamines are a mystic quality to the scientist as well.

One 1921 definition of vitamins. Nearly a decade after scientist Casimir Funk labeled those curious nutritional substances, each vitamin was known basically by the fact that its absence produced a certain disease such as scurvy or polyneuritis.[1] Elusive as these elements were, they captured the imagination and attention of many in the scientific community and among the general public in the interwar period. Granted, little was known about their structure or about the way they worked in the body, but the science of vitamins held out the promise of great benefits. It was this promise, the aura of science, that pharmaceutical companies used to create a new market; it was the promise of science and the aura of science that convinced consumers to embrace these new products.

It is difficult to measure directly the level of popular knowledge. But anecdotal evidence of the public's passion for vitamins abounded during this period. Consumers quickly made use of discoveries in the nutritional sciences. In fact, some critics despaired at the rapidity with which middle-class consumers altered their buying habits. They complained that women in particular had been carried away in their enthusiasm for vitamins. In 1937, one exposé of the pharmaceutical industry contended that "not so long ago the word [vitamins] was unknown to all but the learned. Today, any serious mother is ashamed if she can't discuss vitamins with the greatest of ease. Probably more than one new mother has startled her husband by mumbling in her sleep: 'Milk for vitamin A . . . vegetables for vitamin B . . . oranges for vitamin C . . . and for rare vitamin D baby must have cod-liver oil.'"[2] Vitamins were to be found everywhere: occurring naturally in food, they also appeared in pills and tonics; they enriched flour, were added to soap, and fortified candy.[3] The wealth of correspondence about vitamins in magazines such as *Good Housekeeping* and *Hygeia* suggested the extent of the public's interest. In their letters, readers often expressed concern and confusion over recent announcements in nutritional science. Reading conflicting scientific claims about the beneficial effects of vitamins did not lead them to reject science, however. Rather they asked editors for clarification about scientific claims and about products.

Advertisers swiftly incorporated the public's fascination with vitamins into promotional campaigns; an incredible array of products was championed using the rhetoric of science. Ovaltine was "rich in essential food elements and growth-promoting vitamines," boasted one advertisement.[4] Mothers can serve "Healthful Meals of full Vitamin Content" announced a Kitchen Craft Waterless Cooker promotion. (Figure 1-1).[5] "Children get as much Vitamin B from three heaping teaspoonfuls of Chocolate Vitavose as they do from a *whole quart* of milk," explained still another promotion.[6] An advertisement for Bond Bread informed readers that "scientists agree. . . . All Ages need sunshine vitamin-D."[7] The frenzy over vitamins ranged beyond food products: a cosmetic advertisement proclaimed, "At last a way has been found to feed Vitamin D direct through the pores of the skin . . . with Vita-Ray Cream."[8] And, it extended to nonhuman animals: "O, what would life be without Vitamin D?" queried a dog in an adver-

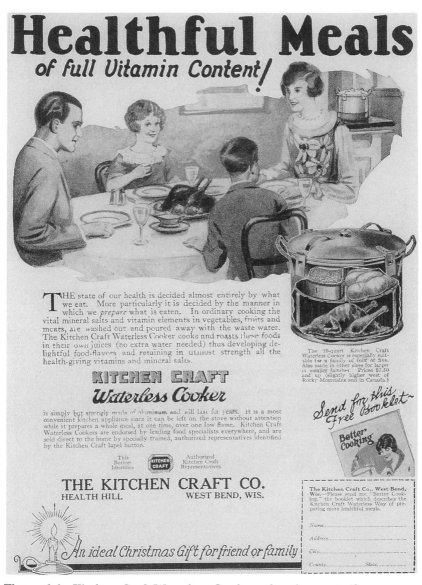

**Figure 1-1:** Kitchen Craft Waterless Cooker advertisement. (Source: *Hygeia*, December 1926, p. 7.)

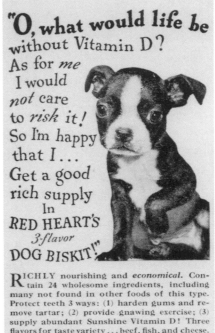

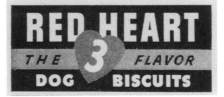

**Figure 1-2:** Red Heart Dog Biscuit advertisement (Source: *Parents' Magazine*, December 1938, p. 96.)

tisement for Red Heart's 3-flavor Dog Biscuits. (Figure 1-2).[9] Amidst all this excitement and foremost among the advertisers who proclaimed the benefits of vitamins were pharmaceutical manufacturers.

The first products widely marketed by vitamin manufacturers were cod-liver oil and its concentrates. In the late eighteenth century cod-liver oil had entered the British Pharmacopeia as a treatment for rheumatism. By the early nineteenth century some physicians also used it to treat gout. Scattered reports of treating cases of rickets with cod-liver oil appeared in nineteenth-century medical literature, but by the end of the century few physicians mentioned the oil, though fishing people and others living close to the sea continued to use it as a tonic. Subsequently, early twentieth-century experiments by researchers McCollum and Davis demonstrated that some fats, including butter fat, egg yolk fat, and cod-liver oil, contain a micronutrient indispensable for the maintenance of life. They named this element fat-soluble A, later vitamin A. By the late 1910s research disclosed the connection between vitamin A deficiency and some eye diseases. Shortly thereafter a comprehensive study by Mellanby proved conclusively that rickets too was a dietary deficiency disease and that certain fats, most notably cod-liver oil, exerted marked preventive and curative effects in cases of rickets. Initially scientists believed that the antirachitic factor was vitamin A, but a few years later McCollum announced the existence of a second fat-soluble vitamin, vitamin D, that was effective against rickets. It was found in cod-liver oil but not butter fat.[10]

The research of Mellanby, McCollum, and others contributed to a renewed interest in the study of rickets. At the same time, nutritional disorders of the bones, seen in Europe particularly in the years following World War I, directed much attention to the cure and prevention of rickets. Admitting that the condition was not a general health problem in the United States, investigators were concerned for specific groups here, especially African Americans and immigrants in eastern urban cities. These groups, it was believed, faced a higher risk for rickets.[11] Soon after this research was published, physicians and other child-health workers increasingly prescribed cod-liver oil. In seeking to eliminate the scourge of rickets, they called for the prophylactic use of cod-liver oil for all children, most especially infants, whether breast-fed or bottle-fed. Child-care educators pronounced cod-liver oil "not a medicine, nor a luxury, but an indispensable food for children of all ages."[12] Mothers all across the country learned the science of vitamins and particularly about the efficacy and necessity of cod-liver oil for children from medical personnel, child-care books and pamphlets, domestic science courses, and manufacturers.

The pervasiveness of science in advertising was so extensive in the 1920s and 1930s that one consumer advocate complained that "a sound knowledge of nutrition is acquired only at some effort and expense, whereas free information of a biased, unscientific nature is thrust upon [the mother] with unrelenting persistency. Every magazine and newspaper flaunts innumerable advertisements of food products and carries articles on diet. Some of these may be sound, but too often they are written with the interests of advertisers in mind."[13] Others observed that the public was receiving its information in the advertising columns of newspapers and magazines where the intent was commercial gain, not science education. They were particularly incensed that "copy writers were especially alert to dramatize the interest in vitamins."[14] Indeed, advertisers knew that science added a certain cachet to their copy and believed that these promotions gained the attention of consumers.

Pharmaceutical companies advertised their vitamins particularly in magazines like *Good Housekeeping, Parents' Magazine,* and *Hygeia.* Such magazines prided themselves on attracting a specific audience: middle-class women, usually mothers. These publications frequently and consciously blurred the line between editorial content and advertising. The advertising department of *Parents' Magazine,* in order to impress current and potential advertisers, used the slogan, "An advertiser's best friend is a mother; a mother's best friend is 'The Parents' Magazine.'"[15] *Hygeia's* column "Among Hygeia Advertisers" directed its readers to specific products and services, claiming that through its advertisements the reader would find "worth while helps and suggestions . . . information of real value to you and your family."[16] The staff of *Good Housekeeping* developed an even closer connection between the magazine and its advertising. It awarded the GH Seal of Approval to products that met standards designed by the Good Housekeeping Bureau. In addition, all products advertised in the magazine, promised the director of the bureau, "whether or not they are within our testing scope, are guaranteed by us on the basis of the claims that are made for them."[17]

In their style as well as their content, advertisements placed by pharmaceutical companies in these magazines employed the latest advertising techniques. Thus, in the 1920s and 1930s advertisements typically made use of the "reason why" and "negative appeal" approaches. As its name suggests, the reason-why advertisement stresses the results of a given purchase more than the actual product itself; in other words, the effect of the advertised product is the reason for purchasing it. A good illustration of this technique is toothpaste advertisements. How often do promoters talk about the ingredients in a dentifrice? They are more likely to depict the romantic potential of using the product. The negative appeal emphasizes the disadvantages of not having purchased the advertised product; in other words, one should buy the product in order to avoid the predicament presented in the advertisement. An example of this today would be advertising scenarios for laundry detergents. Typically the family launderer who does not use the advertised detergent is embarrassed by a stained shirt. The consumer needs to use the correct detergent, such advertisements say, or risk social humiliation. During the interwar period advertisements frequently invoked the reason why and the negative appeal simultaneously. Both techniques share an important characteristic: each uses emotional as well as intellectual arguments to persuade the reader to purchase the product.[18] Pharmaceutical vitamin manufacturers directed their promotions primarily at middle-class women. They presented contemporary scientific claims with reason-why and negative appeal techniques. Their advertisements were characterized by four related themes: fear, hope, guilt, and the contemporary image of motherhood.

The dominant feminine ideology in the 1920s and 1930s was known as "scientific motherhood."[19] The tenets of scientific motherhood placed women in the home where mothers were accorded full responsibility for all things domestic, including, most significantly, the care and raising of children. At the same time, scientific motherhood disparaged women's skills and knowledge and insisted that mothers needed the assistance of medical and scientific experts in order to carry out their maternal duties successfully. Thus scientific motherhood endowed the image of women with both positive and negative attributes: responsibility implies some independence of action and strength, yet the need for assistance suggests dependence and weakness. These conflicting roles created tensions in women's lives.[20] In the vitamin promotions of the pharmaceutical industry, advertising exploited this tension along with the emotions of fear, hope, and guilt.[21]

"Fear" advertisements are the most extreme example of the negative-appeal technique. They warn the reader that dire things will happen, that tragedy will befall her children, unless she buys and uses the product advertised. Scare tactics were familiar from patent medicine and infant food advertisements of the nineteenth and early twentieth centuries.[22] And even in this time period, scare tactics were not unique to vitamin manufacturers. In 1932, worried about declining sales of their high-priced cereal, officers of the Cream of Wheat Corporation hired the advertising agency J. Walter Thompson, which designed a "semiscare appeal to mothers on the dangers of wrong feeding." One advertisement showed a worried-looking little girl in bed. Its headline cautioned: "Little spendthrift of vital energy . . . she has to face double danger now." The copy reminded mothers to "watch the critical years from 1 to 6. Are your children fully protected?" Then this negative appeal was combined with the reason why: the advertisement went on to reassure mothers that Cream of Wheat brought about "steady, *natural* weight gains" and "helps children ward off illness."[23]

The early vitamin advertisements were a little less blatant. They did not target mothers of children with gross vitamin deficiencies such as rickets. They aimed at middle-class mothers who feared the possibility of rickets and other, less specific vitamin deficiency conditions. A typical Squibb promotion from 1926 displayed a picture of its cod-liver oil bottle with the headline "Keep your medicine cabinet out of the shadow of doubt" and the statement "Sturdy young bodies because of it" (Figure 1-3). The copy stressed the vitamin A content of the product, using a reason-why style that emphasized the benefits of cod-liver oil. It then noted that "thousands of children—and grown people too—go unscathed through the harshest winters because of the protection of

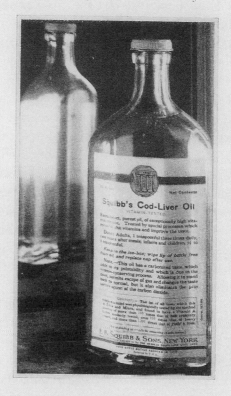

## Sturdy young bodies because of it

THOUSANDS of children—and grown people too—go unscathed through the harshest winters because of the protection of good cod-liver oil. And not only go unscathed, but *glow with increased health* because of its restorative, growth-promoting vitamins.

For good cod-liver oil is the richest known source of the important fat soluble vitamins—and the least expensive. One single pint of Squibb's Cod-Liver Oil is richer in Vitamin A than 1200 pints of grade A whole milk; than one hundred pounds of the best creamery butter!

The vitamins contained in cod-liver oil are especially important for children. They assure normal development of bone and tooth structure.

And Squibb's Cod-Liver Oil is *more palatable*. The special Squibb process insures that. It also insures that the oil will contain its full vitamin content when it reaches you. At drug stores.

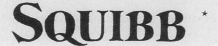

**Figure 1-3:** Squibb's Cod-Liver Oil advertisement. (Source: *Good Housekeeping*, December 1926, p. 249.)

good cod-liver oil."[24] Subtle nods to the negative-appeal style included the headline and the insinuation that mothers who did not use Squibb's Cod-Liver Oil were destined to have sickly children. But on the whole, the tone of this and similar vitamin advertisements of the time was quite positive.

A few months later, however, advertisements for Squibb's Cod-Liver Oil began to exhibit a different quality (Figure 1-4). Here was a reason-why advertisement based primarily on the fear of negative appeal: even the healthiest-looking babies may be developing a deficiency disease.[25] Modern science and medicine have made it clear that mother could no longer trust her own eyes: "Inside, where it can't be seen, the damage starts! A defective development of the bone structure so insidious that it is more than likely to touch even the well-cared-for baby in intelligent modern homes!" A few years later H. A. Metz Laboratories insisted "They Need It NOW," warning mothers that "the ordinary diet is frequently deficient in this essential principle," the sunlight vitamin (Figure 1-5).[26] In a series of advertisements for McKesson's Cod Liver Oil, the company of McKesson and Robbins asked mothers, "Will this war put him 'out of action'? Or will he capture good health—sturdy bones, sound teeth, a straight back?" Furthermore, the copy explained ominously, "It is a war without a roar of cannon—and without quarter! Its very silence makes it sinister."[27]

Yet in the gloomy situations these advertisements depicted, all is not lost: there was hope for the beleaguered mother. In each case, readers learned that conscientious mothers could ward off these threats to their children. "Careful mothers everywhere are using Squibb's Cod-Liver Oil," announced one advertisement (Figure 1-4). "The use of Oscodal protects against rickets," another reassured mothers (Figure 1-5). (Interestingly, "Among Hygeia Advertisers" highlighted this Oscodal advertisement with the comment that "you respect that sort of an advertisement.")[28] "Tide him over the dangerous indoor days—with their lack of sunshine—by giving McKesson's High Potency Cod Liver Oil," counseled still another advertisement.[29]

This mothers' hope was often based on a scientific discovery or

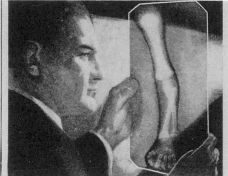

**Figure 1-4:** Squibb's Cod-Liver Oil advertisement. (Source: *Good Housekeeping*, December 1926, p. 249.)

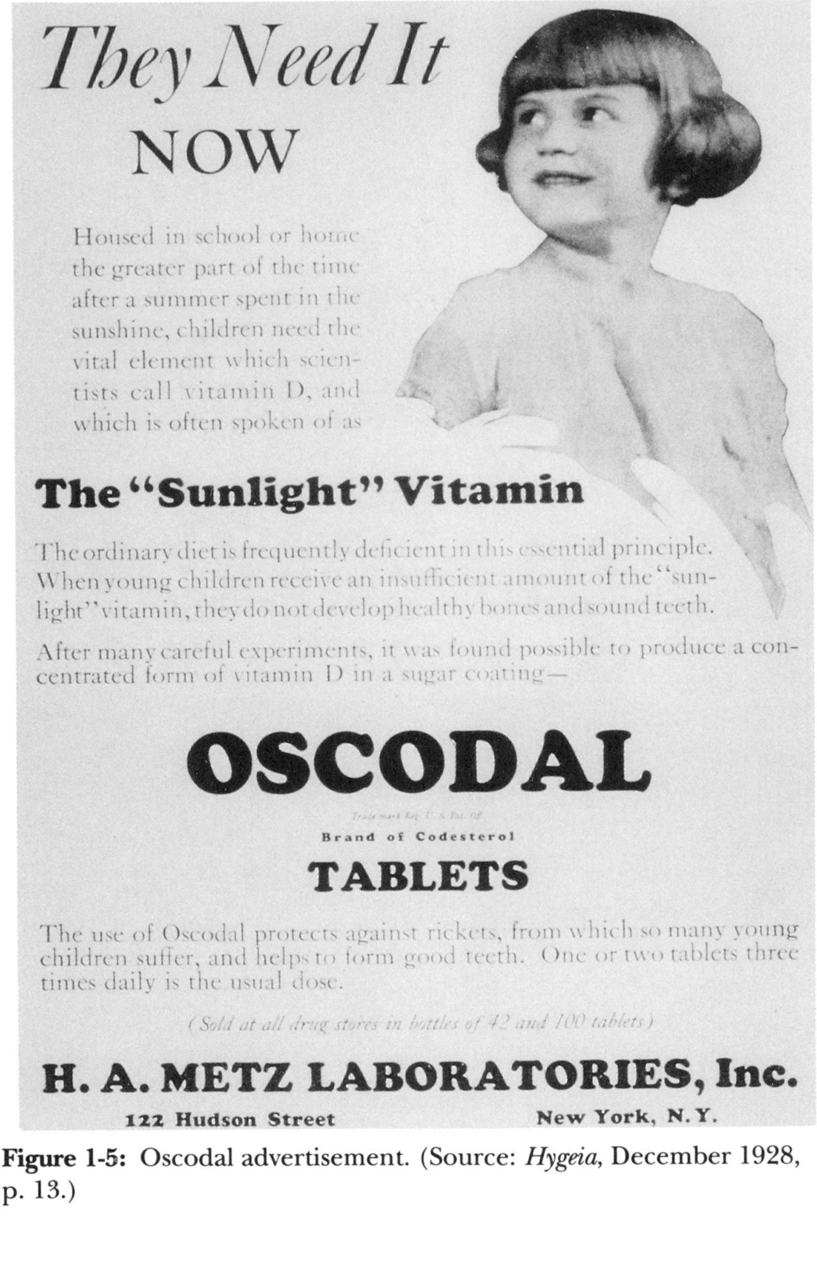

**Figure 1-5:** Oscodal advertisement. (Source: *Hygeia*, December 1928, p. 13.)

on medical expertise. Using the aura of science in advertising was not entirely new nor unique with vitamin manufacturers. But in the twentieth century, advertisements for an increasing number of products more frequently invoked scientific and medical authority. For example, in 1932—in the depths of the Great Depression—the J. Walter Thompson Agency put on a $1 million campaign for the Pineapple Producers Cooperative. Advertisements for canned pineapple in magazines such as *Hygeia* and the *Saturday Evening Post* informed consumers that "research has shown that this one delightful and inexpensive fruit contributes a great number of known dietetic values. . . . It is a good source of vitamins A, B and C."[30] In another advertising campaign to bolster sagging sales, General Mills emphasized that "science reveals why bread is our outstanding energy food."[31]

Similarly, cod-liver oil advertisements delivered the message, either subtly or not so subtly, that scientific and medical authorities recommended cod-liver oil for children. Consequently, if and only if a mother gave her children cod-liver oil could she insure the health of her children. Only with cod-liver oil could she be confident that they would be sick less often and that their bones would develop healthfully. Thus, "children need the vital element which scientists call vitamin D" (Figure 1–5). "It is now scientifically established that sound bones and teeth cannot be formed unless a certain food factor is adequately supplied," warned a Squibb advertisement. "Doctors say a startling percentage of babies' X-ray pictures show failure of bones to grow perfectly," but the advertisement gave the reassurance that doctors knew cod-liver oil would solve the problem (Figure 1–4).

Though fear and later guilt dominated vitamin advertising in the 1920s and 1930s, some of the industry's promotions featured more positive images. In effect they drew on the eminence of science and medicine to promise the reader a fuller, better life if she purchased the product. This genre of advertising included testimonials, such as those for Nason's Cod Liver Oil, headlined "Byrd Antarctic Expedition."[32] Also popular were pictures of happy smiling mothers and babies with captions such as "Everything turned out just as the doctor said—my baby has such *a well shaped head,* such *a fine full chest*" from a Squibb's Cod-Liver Oil advertisement[33] and a chubby smiling baby with the headline, "My Doctor Prescribed Abbott's Cod Liver Oil."[34] This style of advertising highlighted the benefits to be realized when mothers followed the precepts of science and medical experts.

In the 1930s, a new version of the negative-appeal approach appeared in advertising promotions: the fear-provoking situation arose as a direct result of the mother's neglect or uninformed action. In such advertisements, once again, scientific or medical expertise would save the mother from her errors. The clearest example of this type of advertising was a Lysol promotion. Dominating the advertisement was a photograph of a little girl in a crib, her mother and a physician looking very worried.[35] The headline read, "Madam, *you are to blame!*" The copy went on to explain: "She'd have given her right hand to keep her baby well . . . yet that very hand may have caused the illness. And Lysol might have *prevented* it." Apparently the child was ill because the mother did not know the difference between "ordinary house" clean and "the *medical* meaning of cleanliness."

Vitamin advertisements often questioned the mother's knowledge of nutrition and child care, blaming the mother for not knowing the correct dietary supplements to feed her children. "No mother would willingly deny her baby the chance to develop a well-knit frame or a fine set of teeth . . . yet many mothers make this mistake without knowing it!" admonished a Squibb's Cod-Liver Oil advertisement.[36] An advertisement for Whites' Cod Liver Oil Concentrate queried: "Do you know why the winter months are called the danger months? Do you know that science has discovered that the lowered resistance to disease during these months is a direct result of the scarcity in our winter diet of the twin Vitamins A and D—that in winter even the common food sources of these precious vitamins often lack the health giving elements they so abundantly furnish in summer?" The obvious implication was that the reader lacked this vital scientific knowledge and that therefore she was guilty of poor mothering.[37] An advertisement promoting Squibb Adex Tablets-10 D, a vitamin supplement, presented a sketch of a little girl entering school and in the copy explained that "Scarlet fever left Joan hard of hearing" (Figure 1-6),[38] The copy informed the reader that "with many children complications set in [following a childhood illness], simply because their resistance is low!" The advertisement suggested that Joan was now partially deaf because her mother did not help her build resistance with Squibb Adex Tablets-10 D. Copy such as "Lusty legs and sound even teeth are dependent on your care in winter"[39] and headlines such as "Can you keep *your* child off the 'Casualty list'? Will you help him build strong bones, sound teeth, and a sturdy body this winter?" placed the health and well-being of the child in the mother's hands alone.[40] Also, they strove to make the mother feel guilty if she did not buy and use the product.

The graphics and copy of these advertisements typically worked together to establish in the reader's mind a series of premises. First, the mother was responsible for the health of her child. Second, dire consequences would arise unless the mother provided the child with the advertised product. Third, a mother who did not provide the advertised product was not using the most up-to-date scientific knowledge to raise her child. Fourth, any mother who did not apply the most up-to-date scientific knowledge was irresponsible and would be punished with a sick child. In these promotions, pharmaceutical firms used contemporary advertising techniques that neatly juxtaposed the discoveries of science with emotional appeals to culturally accepted images of motherhood.

From 1926 to 1937 consumption of cod-liver oil grew nearly three-fold, from 1.921 million gallons to 5.790 million gallons:[41] an impressive growth, but one, unfortunately, in which the relative importance of advertising is not easy to assess. The promotional campaigns of the pharmaceutical vitamin manufacturers are only part of the story. Medical personnel, public health workers, and child-care educators all were teaching mothers the latest scientific discoveries in vitamin research, and all were also endorsing the drive to encourage the widespread use of cod-liver oil for children. Nonetheless, it is clear that the industry believed there was a relationship.

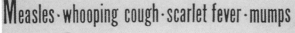

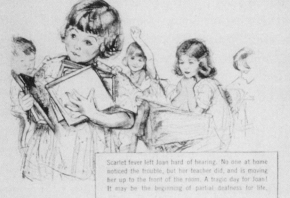

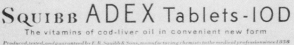

**Figure 1-6:** Squibb Adex Tablets-10 D advertisement. (Source: *Parents' Magazine*, November 1932, p. 43.)

The companies continually expanded their promotional campaigns for all types of vitamin products. One such notable commercial accomplishment was the success of a product called Vitamins Plus. Introduced late in 1937, this combination of vitamins, liver extract, and iron was sold as a beauty aid through department stores.[42] Once again, the target audience for vitamins was middle-class women, not people with gross vitamin deficiencies. In its first six months alone Vitamins Plus spent $150,000 in magazine advertising and $30,000 in newspaper promotions matched by $30,000 of department store funds. This product's primary advertising claims centered on its role as a beauty aid, though the company also proudly announced that Vitamins Plus had been purchased by the Byrd Antarctic Expedition.[43]

Print advertisements for Vitamins Plus emphasized the positive benefits of the product and enjoined women to "Wake up and enjoy life . . . be happily healthy the year 'round . . . With Vitamins Plus, the complete vitamin routine."[44] The company also distributed pamphlets using scientific rhetoric to explain the importance of vitamins in general and Vitamins Plus in particular. Avitaminosis was not a condition only of "poor people" who lacked the financial wherewithal to purchase a healthful diet. No, it could strike anyone, as the brochure "Beauty building from A to G" explained. The Vitamins Plus publication opened with a woman describing the conditions that led her doctor to diagnoses avitaminosis: "People would meet her on the street and say 'You just don't look a *bit* well.' And it was true. Her make-up wouldn't stay put. Her hair came all out of curl ten minutes after it was set. No use to put on nail polish . . . it just chipped right off again."[45] The solution in this negative-appeal advertising was, of course, Vitamins Plus, available at the cosmetic counters of department stores throughout the United States for $2.75 a box containing one month's supply.

Some skeptical consumers asked the Food and Drug Administration if the product was "good and worth the $2.75." According to the FDA, many of the claims for the product "have no adequate scientific basis" and "are not supported by the consensus of reliable medical opinion."[46] The agency felt, however, that given the extent of its regulatory powers, it did "not have a satisfactory basis for legal action."[47] Other queries came to the FDA from the Federal Trade Commission, the agency charged with regulating advertising in this country. At the request of the FTC, the FDA commented on many of the Vitamins Plus claims. Clearly the company and the agency interpreted contemporary scientific research differently. The FDA stated unequivocally, for instance, that "we are familiar with no scientific evidence which indicates that deficiency of vitamins has any bearing of whether make-up will stay put, curl remain in the hair, or nail polish adhere to the finger nails."[48] Soon after, Vitamins Plus, under a stipulation with the FTC, agreed to halt promotions informing consumers that cloudy, lusterless eyes were due to a vitamin A deficiency, that vitamin intake determined the staying power of cosmetics, and that vitamin B removed lactic acid from the bloodstream and consequently eliminated fatigue.[49] Despite this setback, Vitamins Plus enjoyed a long life. Though sales statistics are now unavailable, we do know that by late 1938, a prestigious Manhattan hotel, the Waldorf Astoria, had placed the pills on its breakfast menu. A *New Yorker* cartoon showed the "cigarette girl" at the Stork Club, a popular New York nightclub, selling Vitamins Plus along with cigarettes and cigars.[50] Moreover, the product appeared on store shelves until at least 1960.[51]

Vitamin sales quickly became important to the financial health of the pharmaceutical industry and retail pharmacy. For example, by the 1930s vitamin preparations accounted for between 20 percent and 25 percent of the total sales for Abbott Laboratories; and in the six years after vitamin production began at this company in 1930, the firm's revenues nearly doubled. Pfizer entered the field in the late 1930s and by 1941 vitamins accounted for over 11 percent of the company's sales dollars. Undoubtedly vitamin sales helped these and other pharmaceutical companies through the depression years.[52] Though figures for the value of retail sales varied slightly in different reports, every source documented rapid growth. One *Business Week* article claimed wholesale vitamin sales of $343,000 in 1925 (representing barely 0.1 percent of all drug sales); this figure jumped to $16.11 million a decade later (representing now 5.7 percent of drug sales); in two more years it was $27.1 million (and 8.1 percent). By 1939 the number stood at over $41.6 million, or 11.7 percent of all drug sales. Focusing on retail sales, the total was less than $700,000 in 1925, growing to $32.2 million in 1935, to $54.2 million in 1937, and reaching more than $82.7 million in 1939.[53] The overwhelming proportion of retail vitamin sales occurred in the drugstore. In 1933 the total retail value of vitamins sold in drugstores amounted to about $500,000; by 1937 this figure had grown to $41.8 million.[54]

The public's and the industry's fascination, even obsession, with vitamins continued unabated. As biochemical research provided the data companies needed to develop additional vitamin products, pharmaceutical manufacturers marketed an increasingly diverse range of dietary supplements. Market fragmentation by the 1940s produced products directed toward older consumers and toward infants and children. Today we have special vitamins for infants, like Poly-Vi-Sol, and a variety of products for children, such as E.T.—The Extra-Terrestrial Children's Chewable Vitamins. Adults can choose from among a wide array of products tailored, for example, for their sex (like Within Advanced Multivitamin for Women and Mega-Men), or designed for their lifestyle (like Stresstab High Potency Stress Formula Vitamins), or fitted for their stage of life (such as Eldertonic Vitamin-Mineral Supplement and Stuart Pre-Natal Tablets).[55] Not surprisingly, the sales of the vitamin industry have continued to increase, passing the $1 billion mark in the early 1980s and reaching $4 billion in 1994.[56]

And vitamin manufacturers today still advertise extensively. Contemporary advertisements may be glossier than those of a half-century ago, but they are basically quite similar. As in the 1920s and 1930s, advertisements today draw on culturally accepted images of women and men, placing them in situations recognizable to readers. Most successful advertisements engage the emotions of readers with positive and negative appeals; they play on people's fears and desires and, in the words of one industry analyst, "they're selling hope."[57] The pharmaceutical industry's campaign for cod-liver oil in the 1920s and 1930s reflected contemporary scientific discoveries and established the style and parameters for the next half century of vitamin promotions. Its use of science is intimately intertwined with the development of consumer culture in the United States.

• • • • • • • • • • • • • • • • • • • • • • • • •

# CHAPTER 2

# "To Protect the Interest of the Public"

## Vitamins, Marketing, and Research

The allure of science enhanced the advertising campaigns of the interwar period. Vitamins were mystical and magical. Yet they represented the epitome of modern science and rationality, or so claimed the promotions of vitamin manufacturers. Advertisements did not usually acknowledge the reciprocity between science and commerce. Scientists are not isolated in their laboratories, or immune to the pressures of the marketplace. While advertisements were quick to support their products with the latest scientific advances, the needs of commerce also helped to shape that very research. Scientific researchers, unsurprisingly, were not oblivious to the concerns of manufacturers.

On 12 August 1924, Harry Steenbock, professor of biochemistry at the University of Wisconsin, received an unexpected telegram from a former colleague, Dr. Amy L. Daniels. The wire insisted: "PUBLISH VITAMIN D WORK AT ONCE, DON'T DELAY." In the letter that followed Daniels explained that she had recently learned of another scientist, "a 'pirate,'" who was conducting research on the so-called "anti-rachitic vitamine" and irradiated fats. These were the very subjects of Steenbock's research; he had even submitted a paper on the topic to the *Journal of Biological Chemistry*.[1] The Wisconsin scientist had observed that ultraviolet light enhanced the "growth-promoting and calcifying properties" of some

• • • • • • • • • • • • • • • • • • • • • • • • • • • • • • • • • • • • • • •

ordinary fats, in effect converting them into potent sources for
vitamin D. Steenbock knew his results had commercial application and for this reason had requested that the journal temporarily withhold publication while he applied for a patent.
Daniels's telegram put Steenbock in a quandary. On the one
hand, to establish priority for his work, Steenbook needed to publish quickly. On the other hand, he did not want to publish before
obtaining a patent, a potentially long process. Steenbock released
the paper for publication and also sent a short note about irradiation to *Science*, which published the announcement in the issue of
5 September.[2]

Steenbock initially delayed publication because he feared that
premature announcement of his discovery would ultimately harm
rather than help the public. For him, science should serve the
public good. He wanted a patent before publishing because in his
eyes, a patent could insure the public against unscrupulous merchants. Moreover, it could encourage reputable manufacturers to
develop vitamin D enriched products. At the same time, royalties
generated by the patent could support further research, both his
own and that of others at the University of Wisconsin. Steenbock's
efforts to patent the irradiation process, and his subsequent development of the Wisconsin Alumni Research Foundation to manage the patents, their licenses, and their royalties, generated a
controversy that illuminates the tensions and conflicts that arise
at the intersection of university research and commercial enterprise. It demonstrates the ways in which science in academic laboratories can influence manufacturing. It also shows how the needs
of the marketplace can direct academic research.

The patenting decision reflected concerns and interests that
had shaped and continued to shape Steenbock's life.[3] Brought up
on a family farm in Wisconsin, he understood the importance of
agriculture, particularly dairy farming, to the state's economy.
And, from early in his scientific career he recognized the commercial significance of university research in farming.

Steenbock graduated from the University of Wisconsin in 1908
and was immediately hired as a research assistant by Professor
E. B. Hart, chair of the department of agricultural chemistry. This

job put him in close contact with some of the most creative researchers in biochemistry, including Stephen Babcock and E. V. McCollum. Steenbock's name first appeared on a scientific publication in 1911, for research conducted under Hart and McCollum. In this innovative study, the "single grain ration experiment," four groups of cows were fed carefully controlled diets: one of corn, one of wheat, one of oats, and one a combination of these. The researchers constructed each ration to supply all the known components necessary for healthful growth. According to contemporary chemistry, each ration was analytically identical to the others. Nonetheless the cows differed markedly in their development. At the time, researchers were unable to determine the cause of these differences. But this path-breaking experiment established Steenbock's interest in nutrition research, an interest that later led him to important vitamin discoveries.

As a researcher in agricultural chemistry, Steenbock closely observed a highly successful research department. Hart and Babcock, with the support of Harry L. Russell, formidable dean of the College of Agriculture, had successfully turned university research into practical applications appreciated by the state's farmers.[4] The most visible of these was the invention of the Babcock tester. In 1890 Babcock constructed this mechanism that quickly and accurately measures the butterfat content of milk on the spot. Farmers and cheese makers had long recognized the need for such a device; many of the state's dairy farmers sold their milk directly to cheese factories where the milk's butterfat content set the price. The Babcock tester eliminated the need for highly sophisticated chemical tests or guesswork. Soon after Babcock's announcement, many companies began to manufacture a Babcock tester. Babcock's experience with the tester colored Steenbock's vitamin ventures.

Three and a half decades later, when Steenbock recognized the commercial potential of his earliest vitamin D studies, he was determined to protect the public through patenting. He feared that if he did not patent his irradiation process, someone else would and then would charge industry exorbitant sums for its use. However, if he himself did the patenting, then he could use the authority of the patent to secure the most healthful dissemination of the vitamin process. To bolster his argument, the biochemist offered the recent case of insulin. Researchers in that instance used the control inherent in patenting rights to assure that, in Steenbock's words, "the public is protected against the manufacture of poor preparations and is also protected against extortionate charges and to avoid the possibilities of misusing their discovery which not only would have retarded the further development and use of this product, but would also have resulted in causing untold suffering among diabetic patients."[5] Steenbock had other reasons for pursuing a patent. He was "unwilling to give unscrupulous food and drug venders [sic] the freedom of marketing this or that irradiated product on the basis of preposterous indefensible claims."[6] With a patent he believed that he could supervise licensees and also could oversee their advertising material. In addition, the payment of royalties could bring much-needed research funding to the University of Wisconsin, and thus the results of research would help fund further research. Steenbock had another motive for patenting: to keep the irradiation process out of the hands of the oleomargarine manufacturers.

Margarine had been invented in the nineteenth century, but this cheap butter substitute composed of animal and vegetable fats did not seriously challenge the dairy industry until World War I, when butter was in short supply. Nutrition research demonstrated that oleo lacked vitamin A, an important nutritional element found in butter. Unfortunately, from the dairy farmers' perspective, soon it became possible to correct this deficiency by adding vitamin A during the manufacturing process. A few years later researchers discovered that butter contained vitamin D, which was also missing from oleo. If manufacturers could add vitamin D to margarine, then they could claim that oleo was at least nutritionally equal to butter. Steenbock wanted to protect Wisconsin's dairy industry. Consequently he meant to deny the oleo industry access to an inexpensive source of vitamin D. As he explained his position, "In its broad humanitarian aspects it must be granted that any process which can be used to improve our food and thus improve our health should not be encumbered by restrictions of any kind. But there is another aspect to this matter and that is the effect which such a laissez faire policy would have upon the prosperity of that industry which has contributed most to our nutritional welfare, namely, the dairy industry."[7] Steenbock did not intend to deny American consumers the benefits of readily available vitamin D products, but, according to a colleague, his "primary reason for securing the patent . . . was so that license might be withheld from the oleo interests, to protect Wisconsin's dairy industry."[8]

Despite this interest, many disagreed with Steenbock. In their eyes, patenting by university researchers, particularly those employed at land-grant colleges such as the University of Wisconsin, was most definitely not in the public interest. Inventions and discoveries of faculty and staff at state-financed institutions, they claimed, belonged to the public without restriction. A. J. Glover, influential editor of *Hoard's Dairyman* and a leading spokesperson for the Wisconsin dairy industry, was furious that Steenbock would consider patenting: "Why should the public devote money to discovering new truths only to permit them to be patented and their use determined by some corporations? It seems to me that information discovered by the use of public money belongs to the public and it is difficult for me to understand how such discoveries can be patented and some private corporation determine how they shall be used." He firmly believed that the university had no moral or legal right to take out patents; results of research on the campus belonged to the public.[9]

Glover's position received support from key faculty members, most vocally E. B. Hart, F. B. Morrison, and K. L. Hatch. Early in the century, Babcock had brought Hart to Wisconsin from the U.S. Agricultural Experiment Station in Geneva, New York. Hart quickly became Babcock's disciple. Morrison was a nationally renowned professor of animal husbandry, coauthor of the principal text in the field and also a disciple of Babcock. Hart and Morrison, as well as Babcock himself, believed that the results of university research should be available openly and without limitation to all who need them. Similarly, Hatch, the first director of the university's agricultural extension service, saw university

• • • • • • • • • • • • • • • • • • • • • • • • • • • • • • • • • • • • • •

research as an unrestricted contribution to the state's citizens. Consequently he too vehemently opposed Steenbock's patenting plans.[10]

Even Morrison, who generally opposed patenting, did foresee special circumstances in which research "should be patented if a patent were necessary to protect the discovery against unwise and fraudulent use."[11] Yet he worried that if university researchers were allowed to patent, they might be attracted to commercially feasible projects instead of pure, noncommercial research. Patent opponents feared that both the university and scientific research would be tainted with commercialism.[12] While some saw a difference between receiving royalties from books and from patents, Steenbock believed researchers should be able to protect their findings in the same way that authors copyrighted their ideas.

To justify his patenting efforts, Steenbock frequently retold the story of the Babcock tester. Babcock had refused to patent his invention in order to assure its broad application; in other words, for the good of the public. Subsequently, manufacturers produced cheaply constructed equipment with poorly calibrated test bottles. As a result, this important test was discredited and fell into disuse until states established laboratories to check and standardize the equipment before its sale.[13] To Morrison, the ultimate success of the Babcock tester proved the benefits of not patenting university research.[14] Steenbock focused more on the tester's difficulties; he wanted the control of a patent to avoid such problems.

To some extent Steenbock's fears of "unscrupulous food and drug venders" were realistic. Shortly after Steenbock's announcement, the UltraVol Company attempted to sell an oil that was "activated by a violet ray."[15] A Mr. T. J. Brume claimed to have invented a "superior type" of lamp he wanted to sell to irradiate milk at home.[16] Another enterprising manufacturer, Goodall's Laboratories, produced "Bottled Sunshine," supposedly olive oil exposed to ultra-violet rays. In its advertising the company quoted satisfied customers and experts such as Steenbock. Goodall's sold its product out of the window of a Chicago drug store for $1.25 a bottle (Figure 2-1).[17] And then there was Joseph P. Sereda, who

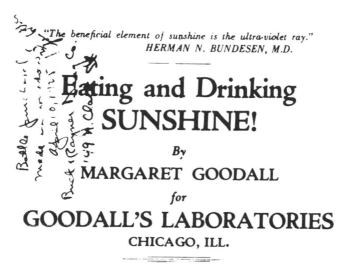

# Eating and Drinking SUNSHINE!

*By*

## MARGARET GOODALL

*for*

# GOODALL'S LABORATORIES

### CHICAGO, ILL.

## BOTTLED SUNSHINE

is now a reality. It is accepted as a proven fact by the foremost authorities in the medical and chemical world, is acknowledged as a specific in some diseases and recognized as of great upbuilding and nutritional value in the treatment of an infinite number of ailments. The condition which is developed in liquids or other matter by the use of the Ultra-Violet Rays, quartz lamp—or manufactured sunlight —has been proven to be the greatest known bone-building, muscle and tissue developing, life giving and vitalizing chemical of the present age. In proof of this statement, allow us to quote from recognized authorities of this country:

HERMAN N. BUNDESEN, M.D., Commissioner Chicago Department of Health, in CHICAGO'S HEALTH BULLETIN, January 3rd, 1925, says:

"Rickets need no longer be considered a terror in infant life.

"Sunshine can now be bottled in other oils as well as in codliver oil, and is effective as an anti-rachitic remedy.

"Children having rickets are more liable to contract pneumonia, and those who do contract pneumonia are far more liable to die. . . .

"In cold climates and in places where the atmosphere is filled with smoke and dust, which render the sun's rays ineffective, science has come to the rescue with an artificial sunlight produced by the mercury quartz lamp. . . . . .

**Figure 2-1:** Bottled Sunshine advertisement, front page. Penciled note reads: "Bottle purchased, made in window, April 10, 1925, Buck and Rayner Drug Co., 149 N. Clark St., $1.25 for bottle." (Source: University of Wisconsin Archives.)

claimed that his "violet-ray machine" cured some eighty different diseases—from abscess through "brain fag" and nervousness to whooping cough and writer's cramp.[18] Cosmetics companies touted the benefits of vitamin D soap. One such product, Cosray, promised to smooth wrinkles, reduce enlarged pores, and eliminate blackheads and pimples.[19]

Dean Russell described the scene that convinced him that the public welfare required patenting of scientific results such as the Steenbock process.

> Shortly after the early public announcement by Dr. Harry Steenbock of his discovery . . . the writer was passing a drug store window in Chicago where a curious crowd was watching a demonstration.
>
> A mazda lamp was shining on a rotating glass plate which was covered with a film of oil that was dripping in a tiny stream from a reservoir above and was being collected in a trough that caught the oil as it flowed off the edge of the rotating plate. The oil was being bottled and the demonstrator was busily engaged in disposing of his cotton seed product to the side walk crowd at a handsome price, making the claim that this product was imbued with wonderful healing properties derived from the electric lamp.[20]

A patent would not prevent all fraudulent use of the process or its name. Yet Steenbock continued to believe that he should patent his work. Only with a patent, the professor insisted, could he exert some control over ethical manufacturers and in some means at least protect the public.

A series of perplexing problems faced Steenbock once he had decided to patent. To begin with, the application process took four frustrating years as the Patent Office raised objection after objection. And Steenbock's troubles did not end once he had acquired his four patents (the first granted in 1928, two more in 1932, and the last in 1936).[21] Then he had to worry about how "to administer the results of research as well as to protect research."[22] Someone had to evaluate license applications, supervise licensees, defend against patent infringements, and manage the funds generated from the royalties. Even before the first patent was granted, Steenbock knew he could not handle all these administrative details himself. Moreover, he felt that as a scientist he needed to distance himself from the commercial, profit-making aspects of the patent. He needed to stand aloof as the scientist, not the merchant.

His first thought was to assign the patents to the university. Such an arrangement, he believed, could profit the public, the manufacturing sector, and the university research community. Eager to benefit the public, the university would be liberal in granting licenses; anxious to avoid costly litigation, industry would be willing to pay royalties, monies that in turn would fund research on the campus. Such an arrangement would protect the consumer and insure that the "public can be served adequately without exploitation and automatically such grants will, to a large extent, protect the public against the charlatan who is always sure to appear with impossible and unwarranted claims."[23]

However, years earlier Steenbock had attempted to assign a patent to the university. He had offered a chemical process that he had developed to produce a highly concentrated form of vitamin A. The UW Board of Regents engaged a legal firm to draw up the patent claim. Evidently, neither the Board nor the law firm saw any urgency and so matters moved slowly. At about the same time, the oleo interests established a fellowship to study the vitamin A process. Believing that these researchers would apply for a patent themselves, the university's lawyers abandoned their efforts. Steenbock was extremely disappointed.[24]

Though frustrated by this experience, Steenbock still felt that he should offer the irradiation process to the university.[25] Once again the University of Wisconsin Board of Regents was slow to act, and, as Steenbock recalled later, "I had to admit that I lost an opportunity to patent my vitamin A discoveries by the dilatory action of the Regents, and that again I could see little or no progress to my request for action [on the vitamin D patent]."[26] Evidently, the UW Board was, at least in part, reluctant for a public institution to enter into a "speculative venture," unless Steenbock would guarantee repayment of any university funds invested.[27] The biochemist was in no financial position to make such a pledge, but he continued to believe that patenting was essential.[28]

Thwarted by the inaction of the board, Steenbock developed a different solution to the sticky problem of patent management. In 1921, two Chicagoans, William Hoskins, a consulting chemist, and Russell Wiles, a patent lawyer, proposed a corporation plan that completely separated the commercial and academic aspects of the situation. Hoskins and Wiles felt strongly that no educational institution could run a successful, efficient business. Instead there should be an independent organization, directed by friends of the university. With this structure, business matters would not concern or distract the university from its educational mandate; yet academe could reap the rewards of a well-managed patent whose royalties would pay for other scientific work. Steenbock never specifically credited Hoskins and Wiles for their idea; but his correspondence strongly suggests that their plan influenced him. In the spring of 1924, Steenbock visited Carl Miner, a Chicago consulting chemist, about pending patent problems. Miner knew Hoskins and Wiles and evidently told Steenbock about the proposal. When the Wisconsin Board of Regents made it clear that they were not interested in handling the Steenbock patent, the researcher discussed the Hoskins/Wiles plan with Dean Russell and Charles Slichter, dean of the UW Graduate School. Both men were excited about the idea. Slichter contacted several alumni who he knew were interested in the future of the school. He persuaded them to create a separate corporation to handle university patents, the Wisconsin Alumni Research Foundation (WARF).[29]

WARF was specifically designed to administer patents for the university's faculty and staff, starting with the Steenbock patents. The foundation was legally and financially independent of the university. The working ties were close, as WARF transferred funds to the university's already established research committee. But the committee, not WARF, selected the projects to be funded. WARF acted as an interface between research (a function of the university) and commerce (a function of industry). WARF, not the professor, granted licenses under the so-called Steenbock patents. The foundation's emblem, not the professor's signature, graced advertisements announcing the vitamin D potency of irradiated products. The foundation also constructed a laboratory that

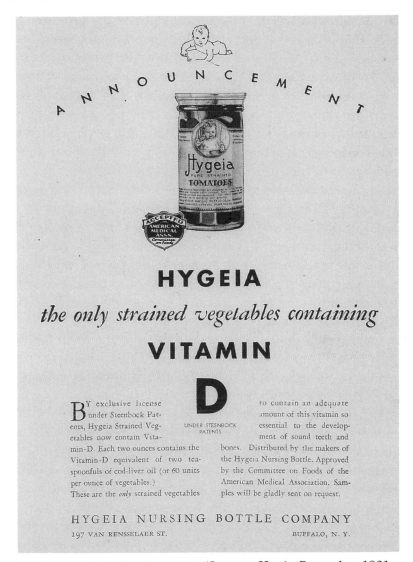

**Figure 2-2:** Hygeia advertisement. (Source: *Hygeia*, December 1931, p. 1168.)

tested the potency of irradiated products to insure that items using the WARF logo met the standards outlined in their contracts. WARF was the focal point of patent management. However, Steenbock did not simply step aside. He worked hand in hand with WARF, especially during its formative years in the 1920s and

1930s. So intricate was the connection between the professor and the foundation that it is very difficult to separate out Steenbock's role from that of WARF trustees or the WARF laboratory. Moreover, WARF, and often Steenbock personally, oversaw the advertising campaigns of manufacturers licensed under the Steenbock patents to assure that companies did not make unwarranted claims and promises (Figure 2-2). WARF even produced its own public service advertisements to educate the public about vitamin D and irradiated products (Figure 2-3).

Steenbock had correctly foreseen the commercial potential of his vitamin D research. One of the first manufacturers to approach Steenbock was Quaker Oats. Studies had demonstrated that dental caries seemed common in countries and areas where oatmeal was widely consumed. Moreover, nutritional experiments had shown convincingly that test animals fed oatmeal exclusively were more likely to develop rickets. Consequently, as early as June 1925, representatives of the company visited the university to discuss with Steenbock this "greatest discovery yet made in the field of nutrition." They wanted a contract with the professor for the rights to use his process for cereal products and they offered to fund further research in this area.[30]

WARF drew up a contract with Quaker Oats in February 1927, even before Steenbock had been granted his first patent. The biochemist was uncomfortable about granting any manufacturer an exclusive contract. Yet Steenbock understood that the company needed a promise of exclusivity before embarking on the costly construction and testing of irradiation equipment. In fact, he used just such a situation to argue for patenting. Before investing heavily in product development, companies needed to be assured that other firms could not just copy their processes and undersell the developers themselves. WARF granted Quaker Oats exclusive use of the process for their products until 1940. WARF also recognized the expense of designing, constructing, and testing new technology; consequently, the contract limited the firm's initial royalties to $5,000 a year. However, once the company began marketing irradiated products, the royalty schedule increased first to $25,000, then to $35,000, and afterward to $60,000 a year.[31] Clearly,

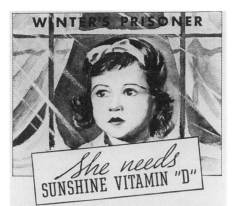

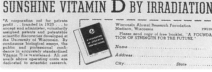

Your baby! There is nothing you wouldn't do to give her the straight, sturdy legs, strong back and sound, even teeth that are her a right to have. Perhaps you have been depending upon the sun to provide the body-building Sunshine Vitamin D she needs to insure a sound bone structure.

*But the sun's Vitamin D benefits become less and less as winter grips the land!* The precious ultra-violet rays are *only one-eighth* as beneficial as in summer. Hours of sunlight are shorter. Children are much indoors. Clouds, smoke, clothing—all these halt the beneficial rays.

*What To Do About It*

To safeguard *your* children against this lack of Vitamin D to help assure them of a foundation of strong, straight bones, of fine, even teeth—do as physicians encourage mothers to do: Serve foods enriched with sunshine Vitamin D—*irradiated* foods ! Through the Steenbock Process, milk, cereals and other foods, as well as pharmaceuticals which your doctor can prescribe, are made rich in Vitamin D through exposure to ultra-violet rays.

Foundation-licensed products— carefully selected for wholesomeness, availability and low cost—contribute definite benefits. The process used is patented to insure exact and dependable scientific control, to help give *your* child a sound "foundation for the future." Send the coupon for free booklet, "A FOUNDATION OF STRENGTH FOR THE FUTURE." *Wisconsin Alumni Research Foundation,* Madison, Wisconsin.*

*Ask for These Products*

You can identify Foundation-licensed products by the word Irradiated and by the reference on the label to the Wisconsin Alumni Research Foundation.

Irradiated Evaporated Milk is available in every part of the United States and Canada, and in many other countries.

Irradiated Vitamin D fluid milk is sold in most large and many smaller cities.

Metabolized Vitamin D fluid milk is supplied in nearly 300 cities.

Other Vitamin D-enriched foods include: Cocomalt; Dryco powdered milk; Ovaltine; Fleischmann's Irradiated Foil Yeast; Quaker Farina, Muffets whole wheat biscuits, and Quaker and Mother's rolled Oats; Sanied Flour.

Irradiated Vitamin D pharmaceutical products are generally prescribed by physicians.

## SUNSHINE VITAMIN D BY IRRADIATION

*A corporation not for private profit . . . founded in 1925 . . . to accept and administer, voluntarily assigned patents and patentable scientific discoveries developed at the University of Wisconsin. By continuous biological assays, the public and professional confidence in accurately standardized Vitamin D is maintained. All net avails above operating costs are dedicated to scientific research.

Wisconsin Alumni Research Foundation
Madison, Wisconsin                                         PM1236

Please send copy of free booklet, "A FOUNDATION OF STRENGTH FOR THE FUTURE."

Name ...........................................

Address .......................................

City ..................... State ...........

**Figure 2-3:** Wisconsin Alumni Research Foundation advertisement. (Source: *Parents' Magazine,* December 1936, p. 60.)

the contract represented a compromise between Steenbock's idealism and the commercial realities of the market place.

Other manufacturers recognized that irradiated products could produce more palatable, more attractive forms of vitamin D than the popularly prescribed cod-liver oil.[32] Despite its undoubted curative and preventive benefits, cod-liver oil had a major disadvantage: it tasted awful. Alert manufacturers recognized the possibilities of advertising irradiated products that were anti-rachitic and more appetizing than cod-liver oil.

Only a few months after publication of his early work in 1924, Steenbock was approached by Eli Lilly, Abbott Laboratories, and other pharmaceutical houses. At that time, the biochemist had felt that talk of the development of vitamin D supplements was premature. However, by 1928 he had concluded that several pharmaceutical houses were probably using his irradiation process without license or control. Subsequently WARF entered into negotiations with four firms (Abbott Laboratories, Mead Johnson, Parke-Davis, and Winthrop Chemical Co.) in order to draw up a mutually advantageous contract, one that would insure WARF royalties and control over the production of the new vitamin D substance named Viosterol (actually irradiated ergosterol) and that would afford the companies protection from competition. E. R. Squibb was also very anxious to gain a license. As the largest producer of cod-liver oil in the country, the company stood to lose a great deal if it were excluded from the negotiations. Squibb was so anxious to be licensed that it agreed to the royalties demanded by WARF, though the company executives considered the price too high. By March 1929, differences between the companies and WARF were resolved and the foundation granted licenses to all five companies.[33]

Other pharmaceutical companies also sought a license from WARF. In turning down the request of one drug company in 1929, Steenbock explained that the five licensees would "be able to furnish the requirements of the trade and made supervision of the quality of the product manufactured [Viosterol] relatively simple."[34] Steenbock made sure that the item in the drug store complied with the standards set out in the licensing contract. First his own laboratory and later a WARF laboratory periodically tested samples bought in local drugstores.[35] Steenbock also took a direct interest in the advertising campaigns of the licensed pharmaceutical companies.[36]

Like the pharmaceutical companies and Quaker Oats, a multitude of other food manufacturers were anxious to irradiate their products. Vitamins were receiving much attention in the press and irradiation was a relatively simple way to enhance the advertising potency of food products. Interested firms ranged from the Anheuser Busch brewery and Fleischmann's, producer of yeast, to C. E. Wheelock, manufacturer of jams and jellies, and Bottled Beverages, Inc., of Cleveland, Ohio, who in 1929 was "working on a chocolate drink with the idea of introducing Vitamine 'D' thru irradiated argosterol [*sic*]. This, of course, will make a chocolate drink worthwhile to sell to the public school children and other kiddies thruout the land."[37] Most of the many, many letters of inquiry met with rejection. Steenbock explained that WARF issued licenses to only "the most important food products such as milk, cereal, fats, and the like" in order that researchers could "ascertain the reaction of the public" and "have available exact data on the physiological effect of the product on human nutrition."[38] Several companies were able to work out satisfactory licensing contracts with WARF. The oleo industry, though, was shut out.

When it came to preserving Wisconsin's dairy industry, even faculty members who disapproved of patenting university research agreed with Steenbock. Denying an irradiation license to oleomargarine, these professors believed, was like the principle of protective tariffs, "simply as a protection of Wisconsin's main agricultural industry" and a protection of the university. Explained Prof. Morrison to Dean Russell as early as 1925, "If human suffering could be alleviated only by licensing the irradiation of oleo margarine, then I will agree that we would be remiss in our duty if we opposed it, even though it might be detrimental to the financial welfare of the College. However, it is not necessary for people to secure the anti-rachitic property of oleomargarine."[39] For nearly twenty years, Steenbock and WARF agreed with this rationale and refused oleomargarine licensing. By 1942, though, the situation had altered significantly. New processes had been developed that could produce more palatable vitamin D products, sometimes at less expense than direct irradiation. Therefore, Steenbock felt, his process no longer monopolized the synthetic vitamin D field and consequently WARF was no longer in any position to protect the butter industry.[40]

Steenbock and WARF were very aware of the development of

alternative sources. During the 1930s, the problem of fluid milk presented a significant commercial challenge. Various milk companies and creameries inquired about the possibility of vitamin D milk shortly after Steenbock's initial announcement, but he did not turn his attention to the problem until sometime after 1930. Several different methods could be used to produce milk rich in vitamin D. Steenbock preferred his method of direct irradiation of fluid milk. Under the auspices of WARF a few manufacturers of dairy equipment developed machinery that produced irradiated vitamin D milk with no off-taste. By 1934 WARF was licensing large dairies to produce this milk. Irradiated milk soon confronted stiff competition from milk fortified with a vitamin D concentrate called Vitex, produced by the National Oil Products Company. The lower cost of Vitex milk gave it the edge with many dairies. Aware of the importance of vitamin D milk both for the health of the public and for its own economic health, WARF financed the development of its own vitamin D concentrate for milk, UVO, which was introduced into New York in 1937 "as a defensive measure in competition with Vitex."[41]

This example should not suggest that Steenbock or even WARF cared only for monetary gain. The motivations of researchers and the foundation were much more complex. On the one side, the expense of the irradiation process raised the price of milk; on the other side, concentrates were so cheap that there was no difference in price between vitamin D milk and unfortified milk. "Our original goal in the fluid milk field," the trustees reminded themselves in 1936, "was to secure the treatment of the milk of the masses. We will never realize this on the basis of a premium milk." While concerned for WARF's financial health, the WARF board of trustees also considered its social responsibilities.[42]

By the 1940s WARF was firmly established and financially secure. Steenbock's dream had become reality. The chemist had demanded patenting to protect the public from fraud and quackery; he had designed WARF to distance himself from the taint of commercialism. Yet market forces shaped WARF. To avoid any charge of commercialization, Steenbock refused to accept any of the royalties paid to WARF. However, the WARF board of trustees insisted that he receive some remuneration. They argued that if Steenbock received nothing from the foundation for his patents, then other faculty might be unwilling to turn their patents over to WARF. Finally the board of trustees forced Steenbock to accept 15 percent of the net income generated from his patents; WARF invested the remaining 85 percent.[43]

Though at first unwilling to accept any royalties, over the years Steenbock came to appreciate the money as a source for funding additional research. In other ways, too, Steenbock's views changed under the press of commercial considerations. His response to Mr. A.V.H. Mory, director of the Technical Bureau of the Biscuit & Cracker Manufacturers' Association, was typical of his views in the early 1920s. Mory had inquired about the possibility of producing a "vitamine" cracker (this before Steenbock's vitamin D work). Steenbock replied that he knew "nothing of the manufacture of crackers." He pointedly dissociated himself from the commercial aspects of vitamin research and suggested that manufacturing was "a problem of your consulting chemist and technologists rather than of one who is interested in the problems related to vitamines from the scientific standpoint."[44] Soon he recognized how difficult it would be to separate basic and applied research. "Obviously before commercial use can be made of the findings to date," he wrote an executive of the Postum Cereal Company in 1924, "extensive experiments will have to be carried out to make its commercial use economically practical. We are prosecuting such experiments as rapidly as possible."[45] With vitamin D milk and so many other instances, Steenbock found himself drawn more and more into the commercial side of ultraviolet irradiation.

Helping manufacturers develop effective irradiation processes was one way Steenbock carried forth his, and WARF's, mission to protect the consumer. In addition he, and WARF, bought and tested licensed irradiated products in their own laboratory to insure their uniformity and reliability. As more and more manufacturers enriched their products with vitamin D, whether using the Steenbock process or another form of supplement, Steenbock became less committed to protecting the public from such fortified foods. The April 1936 issue of *Modern Brewer* contained an article extolling the virtues of vitamin D beer, just the sort of a "frivolous" product that Steenbock had ridiculed earlier. WARF's board considered demanding that the magazine admit "the fallacy of incorporating Vitamin D in beer." The professor advised against any action. By the late 1930s, Steenbock was less committed to his role as protector of the public and more savvy about the commercial world. As he viewed the case of vitamin D beer,

> In the past in the absence of competition from other sources of vitamin D and in the absence of the slightest attempts on the part of governmental control, it was perfectly proper for the Foundation to state succinctly what responsibilities it was assuming and to what extent it was actively protecting the public. But at the present time there is no question but that the policy of functioning as a protecting agent is rapidly being undermined. . . . it no longer is advisable for the Foundation to assume an ultra-idealistic attitude. In other works, if the public should demand vitamin D in its beer, there is no reason why the Foundation should not provide it—because it may do some good and it most certainly will not do any harm.[46]

Since its establishment in 1925, the foundation had changed also. A pioneer among nonprofit university-affiliated patent-management agencies, WARF had become a model emulated throughout the United States. By 1956 there were more than fifty similar, separately incorporated organizations.[47] From the beginning WARF's trustees, primarily business people and lawyers working on a volunteer basis, conducted nearly all the business of the foundation. But soon the phenomenal success of the Steenbock patents demanded more professional administration. The problem of patent litigation plagued the foundation. As patents were granted, the task of reviewing license applications grew; so did the job of negotiating royalties and monitoring payments. The WARF laboratory kept busy testing licensed products to assure they met foundation standards. Similarly, WARF personnel, and often Steenbock, reviewed and rewrote advertisements for vitamin D products licensed by WARF. These tasks are one side of patent management. WARF also handled the investment and disbursement of royalties.[48] With interest in the Steenbock patents high in the 1930s, the royalty fund increased dramatically. The achievements of the Steenbock patents and WARF were so overwhelming that by 1930 Harry L. Russell resigned as dean to become the foundation's first full-time director and to oversee the continued growth and development of WARF.[49]

Still, despite WARF's success, the rationale underlying its development remained in dispute: Should university researchers patent their discoveries? Did patenting represent consumer protection, or should patents be shunned in the name of public interest? WARF continued to face charges of unfair licensing practices.[50] Some felt strongly enough to take direct action; they challenged the patents in court.

In the summer of 1943, a federal appeals court in San Francisco held that Steenbock's patents were invalid. But, it is important to note, the court did not rule on whether a university or researcher could patent a discovery. The court decided on much narrower grounds instead: the irradiation of foods with ultraviolet rays was a natural process; Steenbock had discovered it but not invented it; and, most significantly, as a natural process it could not be patented. WARF continued the court fight for several more years, but all litigation ceased in October 1945 when the Supreme Court refused to review the lower court's ruling; the Steenbock patents were invalidated. Interestingly, the main Steenbock patent, received in 1928, had expired on 13 August 1945. On 11 January 1946, WARF "dedicated to the public" the remaining three U.S. patents.[51]

Was Steenbock wise to patent his process? Were his critics vindicated? Had WARF managed to balance successfully the demands of research funding, public welfare, and commercial growth? Clearly there is no simple answer. True, the patents, while they lasted, gave Steenbock and WARF some control over the commercial use of irradiation. They were able to insist on standards of production and truth in advertising. Also the royalties generated an enviable endowment fund for research at the University of Wisconsin. Still, WARF and Steenbock were, as they had to be, influenced by market considerations. As Steenbock rationalized: "While, of course, there are many questions of scientific interest which could be investigated . . . , there are some which under the circumstances assume more importance than others. Although, of course, it is not our desire to emphasize the practical unduly, yet it appears that there is no reason why certain phases distinctly scientific should not be given preference because of their utilitarian aspect."[52] The development of UVO, the denial of a license to the oleomargarine industry, the licensing of only five pharmaceutical houses, the granting of patents to Quaker Oats—all were decisions informed by the lucrative vitamin market.[53]

The science of vitamins created a conundrum for university researchers. Working in field with momentous commercial potential, they were drawn into the marketplace. Their involvement can be cast in both positive and negative light. On the one hand, scientists such as Steenbock, who worked intimately with the market, emphasized the importance of control.[54] A consistent theme running through his work and writing is his conscious commitment to the public good; he genuinely feared the effects of the uncontrolled application of irradiation. He devoted much of his research to making vitamins more available to the American consumer and to devising more effective irradiation processes. Additionally, he felt responsible for the implementation of irradiation and impelled to monitor the products produced with his patents. Obviously, patenting shaped his laboratory work. Many interpreted the time spent on application development and product testing as "commercialization." It is clear, however, that Steenbock would characterize this work as "humanitarian," as protecting the public.

Those opposed to patenting focused on the money-making aspects of the procedure. They insisted that researchers would follow the demands of the marketplace for new products, rather than the pursuit of pure research. They equated patenting with excessive royalties and, in the 1920s and 1930s, for example, insisted that irradiated products would be much less expensive if manufacturers had no royalties to pay. They pointed to WARF's undeniably large endowment fund as proof of profiteering. Therefore, opponents found that patenting was detrimental to the public good.

Steenbock, the professional scientist, believed that his vitamin discoveries could benefit the American populace. But he was not only a scientist; he was also a faculty member at the University of Wisconsin and a citizen of Wisconsin. As all these and more, Steenbock strove to balance the demands of research, of politics, and of the marketplace. In the professor's hands, the science of vitamins endowed the highly prosperous Wisconsin Alumni Research Foundation and brought university research closer to the commercial world. With vitamins science was removed from the laboratory and placed squarely in the center of American culture and commerce.

• • • • • • • • • • • • • • • • • • • • • • • • • • •

# CHAPTER 3

# "Superior Knowledge"

## Pharmacists, Grocers, Physicians, and Linus Pauling

When people learn that I am writing about the history of vitamins, the first question often asked is: What about Linus Pauling and vitamin C? To many in this country Pauling personifies the issue of vitamins. With the fervor of a convert, Pauling dramatized the vitamin controversy. He and his partisans made clear that there was no single, simple explanation of the data on vitamin C therapy. They capitalized on the very uncertainty about the science of vitamins to raise questions about the authority of professionals and experts in directing our everyday life. The science of vitamins challenged the limits of professional superiority in our consumer society.

Pauling's view of professional authority was very different from that of Harry Steenbock. From the outset of his investigations, Steenbock had portrayed himself as a disinterested scientist, a professional with the expertise and the responsibility to safeguard the American consumer. Only after many decades did he accept his impotency in this area. Others, however, continued to use the mantle of professionalism to claim the high ground for themselves in the world of vitamins. The power and mystery of vitamins were invoked by two very different health-care professions to gain the confidence of the American public. Both pharmacists and physicians used the ambiguity about vitamins to strengthen their professional positions.

Vitamin pills are an enigma. Are they food to be sold in a grocery store or are they drugs dispensed in a pharmacy? Druggists approached middle-class consumers and the courts cloaked in professionalism. They argued that they should be the sole purveyors of vitamin products, which are drugs. Are vitamins preventatives for deficiency diseases or do they work systemically to enhance our health and prolong our lives? Physicians followed Pauling into the public media to persuade American consumers that medical doctors should answer such questions, not nonmedical personnel. Pharmacists and physicians used the very elusiveness of vitamins to define and defend the power and authority of their professions.

From the earliest years of vitamin marketing, vitamins were typically sold in drugstores. Slowly, other retail outlets recognized the economic potential of these products. The target audience for these pills was not the ill, not those who showed signs of gross vitamin deficiency. All agreed sick people should be under the care of a physician. Rather, the goal was to persuade the middle-class consumer, concerned for her general health and the health of her family, to purchase vitamins. By the late 1930s, pharmacists were extremely anxious about the competition from other retailers; their concern focused on grocers. The controversy came to a head in 1939 when the Kroger grocery chain announced very loudly and very publicly that they were selling vitamins.

Though Kroger Grocery and Baking Company was the lightning rod that galvanized concerted and organized opposition of druggists, it was not the first nondrug retailer to market vitamin products. Department stores had been selling Vitamins Plus at their cosmetic counters for several years; by 1939 other products such as Daily Vitamins were also sold as beauty aids. Chain stores such as Woolworth, Kresge, Newberry, and Green all climbed on the vitamin bandwagon with products of their own:[1] and for very good reason, considering the economic potential of vitamins. As early as 1936, a major drugstore publication, *Drug Topics*, estimated that at least one-third of all drug business consisted of vitamin products. Of even greater importance to druggists, vitamins

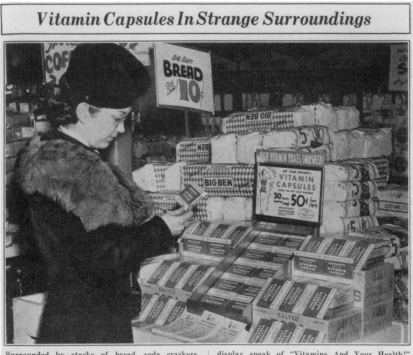

**Vitamin Capsules In Strange Surroundings**

Surrounded by stacks of bread, soda crackers, coffee, sugar is this display of vitamin capsules in a Toledo, Ohio, store of the Kroger Grocery & Baking Company chain. "Get Your Kroger's Vitamin Capsules When You Buy Your Groceries," reads the poster, while leaflets at the base of the display speak of "Vitamins And Your Health!" Soon to join this grocery chain in the selling of vitamins is the Independent Grocers' Alliance whose 5,000 voluntary members, most of them located in the Middle and Far West, will offer capsules beginning May 1. Story in column 4.

**Figure 3-1:** "Vitamin Capsules in Strange Surroundings." (Source: *Drug Topics*, 10 April 1939, p. 3. Reprinted with permission of *Drug Topics*, Medical Economics Publishing, Inc.)

represented 18 percent of all sales in the average drugstore.[2] Pharmacists used professional authority to justify their monopoly over vitamin sales, but they did not deny the financial importance of these products in the pharmacy.

In February 1939, Kroger began the sale of its own "A-B-D-G Vitamin Capsules" with a direct attack on vitamin prices in drugstores (Figure 3-1). Touting the advantages of buying both groceries and vitamins in the same location, advertisements showed an exploding firecracker with the copy: "BANG Go High Prices On Vitamin Capsules." The copy went on to explain: "You need vitamins—plenty of vitamins—to keep yourself in shape. Now you can get them, at amazingly low cost. . . . Take a capsule daily, at a cost of only 1 ⅔ cents!" Quickly the national drugstore and grocery press picked up the unfolding story.[3] Just as quickly, the pharmacy profession responded. Within weeks, the Indiana Board of Pharmacy informed the company's management that only stores they licensed could sell vitamin products. Kroger answered with its own suit. The chain dismissed the board's authority to issue such a regulation. It contended that vitamin capsules were not drugs; they were food.

Over the next several months, Kroger and the board lined up witness after witness in Marion County Superior Court arguing the question: Were vitamins to be classified as food or as drugs?[4] In the company's description, A-B-D-G Vitamin Capsules were composed of "constituent parts and elements of natural food materials essential for normal nutrition [which] are found in varying degrees and quantities in various foods and food products." Its suit claimed that the regulations restricting the sale of vitamin products to licensed drugstores were "arbitrary, capricious, improper and unlawful." Kroger asked the court to rule that the regulation had "no force and effect."

The board and its witnesses defined vitamins differently. To pharmacists, vitamins "constitute drugs or medicine." The board submitted evidence that Kroger agreed with this definition. The court record contained advertising flyers that explained the science of vitamins to consumers. One of them, headed "YOUR VITAMINS/And Your Health!," presented two columns:

| ENOUGH VITAMINS | NOT ENOUGH VITAMINS |
| --- | --- |
| Bright eyes | Dull eyes |
| Good vision | Night blindness |
| Lustrous hair | Dull or falling hair |
| Good bones | Poor bone structure |
| Good teeth | Soft dentine and enamel |
| Fit feeling | Tiredness, irritability |
| Buoyant vitality | Serious deficiency diseases |

Some of the circulars reminded consumers that A-B-D-G Vitamin Capsules were "not intended to give you *all* the vitamins you need," that they were to be used as supplements. Others explained that "not getting enough vitamins regularly will injure your health. Many people are vitamin deficient." And some listed the specific conditions that could arise from vitamin deficiency; for example, insufficient vitamin A could "cause night blindness, dry, scaly skin, poor teeth, lowered resistance to colds, and improper muscular function." Moreover, the board showed that the company had reached out to Indiana physicians, informing them that patients could now buy vitamin supplements at prices lower than those in drugstores. All this, the board claimed, demonstrated that vitamins were not foods and, most tellingly, that Kroger recognized the medicinal value of vitamins.

By 1 December 1939, the court entered its final judgment; it decided against the board and sustained Kroger's contention that vitamins in whatever form were food. Less than four weeks later, the board appealed and asked for a new trial. When this was denied, the board took the case to the state supreme court.

Kroger did not limit its vitamin promotions to the state courts. While the Indiana litigation was winding its way through the judicial system, the company also made its case on the federal level. In the early 1940s, the Food and Drug Administration proposed labeling regulations for "special dietary foods." Kroger filed a brief at those hearings, contending that vitamin products such as A-B-D-G Vitamin Capsules are "foods represented for use in preventing or correcting dietary deficiencies." Furthermore, Kroger positioned itself on the side of public health; its brief pointed out that while Kroger's vitamins were selling for fifty cents a box, the drugstore price was two to five times as much. The company charged that a pharmacy monopoly on vitamins was clearly in the "interests of the drug store trade," but was a "detriment" to the public good. Kroger conceded its own obvious financial interest in unrestricted sales, but the company magnanimously concluded that in this case the company's interests and those of the public coincided.[5] The American Pharmaceutical Association (APhA) and the National Association of Retail Druggists (NARD) did not let Kroger's brief remain unanswered. A few days later, they addressed the hearings. First they claimed that Kroger's brief was not germane. The FDA, according to APhA and NARD, had no authority to determine whether a product was a drug or a food; such determination lay with the Federal Food, Drug and Cosmetics Act of 1938. Secondly, A-B-D-G Vitamin Capsules provided a long list of diseases for which the product was indicated. This labeling, the brief insisted, classified the product as a drug.[6] The hearing was adjourned with no resolution. Due to administrative shifts in the federal regulatory system, the proposed labeling regulations were temporarily set aside.[7]

In answering the threats from grocery chains such as Kroger, pharmaceutical organizations and individual pharmacists designated themselves as professionals with expertise unmatched by grocers and grocery clerks. When pushed, druggists too would sometimes admit that technically vitamins were food and not drugs; still, they would warn, this definition was dangerous when applied to concentrated vitamins. A deficiency of a vitamin results in a deficiency disease; hence, druggists said, vitamin concentrates used in the prevention and treatment of disease should be considered drugs and must be sold only by pharmacists who "are capable of advising the public on their proper use." Pharmacy leaders rapidly recognized that if druggists wanted to retain the profitable vitamin business, then they must emphasize "superior knowledge of the properties and uses of vitamin products." Article after article in the retail drug press reiterated this idea: to preserve and enlarge their vitamin sales pharmacists must present themselves as professionals whose advice could be trusted. With this expertise and the consequent confidence of the customer, druggists could be more effective in vitamin sales than grocers.[8] This theme of professionalism echoed through the decades, even while druggists discussed the profitability of vitamin products. Editorials, in text and cartoon, drove home this point. In 1942 *Drug Topics* affirmed that "vitamins are therapeutic products and should be featured and promoted as such. Once pharmacists go all-out for vitamin business and interpret vitamin preparations in a professionally competent manner, they need not worry even if

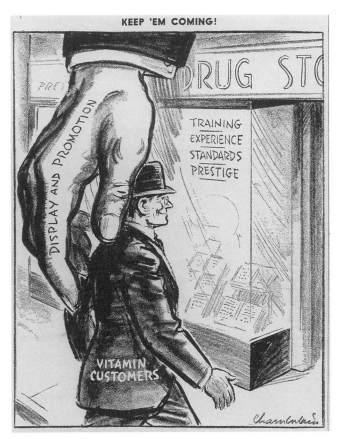

**Figure 3-2:** "Keep 'em coming!" (Source: *Drug Topics*, 25 May 1942, p. 16. Reprinted with permission of *Drug Topics*, Medical Economics Publishing, Inc.)

the courts, reformers, and other yearners go all-out for nutritional hokum"[9] (Figure 3-2).

The extent of pharmacists' professionalism vis-à-vis vitamins is an open question. Were they highly knowledgeable in the details of vitamin deficiency conditions and able prescribers of nutritional supplements? Just how superior were they to grocery clerks? The retailing strategies proposed in the drugstore literature and the practices described by pharmacists suggest that their actual expertise spanned a broad spectrum. The comments of some reflected the contemporary discussions in the medical, sci-

entific, and pharmaceutical press; others did little more than reproduce the language of vitamin advertisements. Regardless of
the pharmacists' actual level of training and knowledge, promotional campaigns to attract and retain customers placed most of
the emphasis on professional image. The science of vitamins enhanced the professional stature of pharmacists. The controversial
nature of vitamins mandated that consumers trust the expertise of
a professional in selecting a vitamin pill.

Meanwhile, the Kroger case continued through the courts with
extensive press attention. It was the first major court test of
Boards' of Pharmacy regulations restricting the sale of vitamin
products to drug stores, but by no means the last. Other states
looked to Indiana for guidance and for indications of how the
judicial system would handle such claims and counterclaims. After its judicial defeats in 1939, the board appealed to the Indiana
Supreme Court. The February 1943 decision was not, however,
what the board had wanted. Rather than clearly defining the extent of the board's authority, the court simply found that the
lower court did not have jurisdiction in the case.[10] This inconclusive resolution sent the board back to redraft their vitamin regulations. In November 1943, it released new rulings that appeared
closer in accord with contemporary thinking. Now vitamin products were classified according to the claims on their labels. Products specified for "the prevention, treatment or cure of disease"
were considered drugs within the meaning of the Indiana pharmacy law, to be sold only by registered pharmacists. Other vitamin
supplement products could be labeled as "Not for Medicinal Use"
and could be sold by those not registered with the Board of Pharmacy.[11]

Other states followed a similar pattern: Boards of Pharmacy
would attempt some restriction on the sale of vitamin products.
The courts and sometimes the legislatures would be brought into
the picture. Representatives of the retail food industry would
claim that vitamins were food and representatives of the pharmacy industry would argue that vitamins were drugs used to prevent and treat diseases. Typically the attorneys involved pointed to
similar cases in other states and repeated each others' arguments.

Then laypersons, judges, and lawmakers would decide: food or drugs? Did one need professional training to sell vitamins? In New Jersey, the courts determined that vitamins and vitamin products were foods; in Minnesota, the attorney general determined that they were drugs. Several states followed the path of Indiana, striking a compromise that permitted the sale of packaged vitamins in nondrug outlets when labeled "not for medical use."[12]

In New York, it was not an individual company or grocer who fought the decision to define vitamins as drugs; rather it was a committee composed of individual retail grocers, the New York State Food Merchants Association, the Supermarket Institute, several large chains, and some vitamin manufacturers. The Board of Pharmacy had asked the state attorney general for an opinion on whether vitamin products could be classified as drugs. The attorney general considered the question in terms of the statutes governing pharmacy education. Since the law recognized items listed in the United States Pharmacopeia (USP), the official homeopathic pharmacopeia, and the national formulary as drugs, and since vitamins A, $B_1$, $B_2$, C, and D were listed, he ruled they were drugs. The law also allowed the board to judge the class of an item by its intended use; that is, if "scientific and professional opinion of those competent and qualified to express the results of research and study" determined that products were intended for "the diagnosis, cure, mitigation, treatment or prevention of disease," then the board had the power to define the items as drugs. The attorney general's opinion went even further: "You are not required to be blind or deaf to the claims of the manufacturers of vitamins so frequently and voluminously advertised to the public."[13] In other words, if manufacturers set their products up as treatments or preventatives, they could no longer argue that these items were foods.

The attorney general's opinion was applauded in pharmacy circles, and the grocers were dismayed. They protested that such a ruling gave druggists a virtually monopoly on a $250 million a year business. The New York State Food Merchants Association estimated that 5,000 of the state's 29,000 grocery stores sold vitamins and the group threatened court action. Other partisans joined the dispute. Benjamin Harrow, professor of biochemistry and an early vitamin researcher, felt compelled to send a letter to the editor of the *New York Times*, in which he deplored the attorney general's decision. Vitamins, he insisted, were "as much a part of our food as protein, fat, carbohydrate, minerals, water and oxygen." They are needed for the normal functioning of the body. They are not drugs because "drugs are not part of our daily food; they are not needed for the normal functions of the body. They are used for a specific purpose—to prevent or overcome various abnormalities, infections, etc."[14] The *New York Times* itself railed against the decision. It editorialized that many other items were in the USP, such as sugar and gelatin, and were not considered drugs; that other products, such as mineral oil, mustard plaster, and surgical gauze were used in treatment, yet they were not drugs. A drug should be defined not by a law but by "a board of competent biochemists."[15] It is significant that both sides of the issue called for expert, professional evaluation of the issue and both used the public interest to support their definition of vitamins as food or drugs. The grocers alleged that public welfare required a free and unrestricted market for vitamins. The pharmacists insisted that this was simply a ruse on the part of grocers who were more interested in sales than public health.[16]

As in Indiana, the resolution in New York State was based on a technicality. The New York State Food Merchants Association sued the Board of Pharmacy, and then the board requested that the court dismiss the complaint. The court denied the motion, explaining that the question was not whether the board had the power to regulate the sale of drugs; the question was, did it have the power to prohibit unlicensed vendors from selling food? If vitamins were food, then the board's restriction amounted to an unconstitutional and unwarranted exercise of power.[17] As in Indiana, the New York debate apparently went no further.

Whether or not they won in the court, druggists knew they had to persuade their customers that professional knowledge counted when it came to vitamins. Frequent stories in the drug-trade literature described how individual pharmacists enhanced their professional aura and how this technique successfully increased vitamin

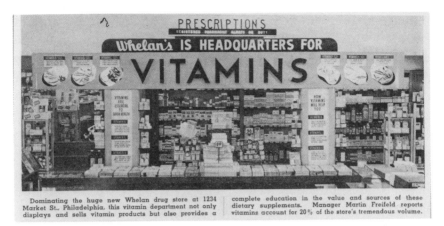

Dominating the huge new Whelan drug store at 1234 Market St., Philadelphia, this vitamin department not only displays and sells vitamin products but also provides a complete education in the value and sources of these dietary supplements. Manager Martin Freifeld reports vitamins account for 20% of the store's tremendous volume.

**Figure 3-3:** Whelan drugstore. (Source: *Drug Topics*, 29 May 1944, p. 43. Reprinted with permission of *Drug Topics*, Medical Economics Publishing, Inc.)

sales (Figure 3-3). Some pharmacists depicted themselves as partners in health care with physicians. Clearly focusing on middle-class consumers in close contact with doctors, Gene Gilmour, proprietor of a drugstore in Lincoln, Nebraska, installed window displays that recommended that customers talk with their physicians before buying vitamin products. This tactic, Gilmour believed, served several purposes. First, it established goodwill for the store with the local medical practitioners, a not incidental benefit for a pharmacy that filled many prescriptions. Second, it created a positive image for the drugstore, an image of reliability. Third, it attracted the customers who had a clear idea of which vitamins they wanted by "impress[ing] the public with the fact that the drug store is the place to buy drugs and kindred items."[18] For Gilmour, this policy established a professional deportment that clearly and consciously differentiated his drugstore from grocery stores and other nondrug outlets.

Other pharmacists walked a fine line between pharmacy and medicine, between advising customers about appropriate vitamin products and usurping the physicians' role to prescribe. In his drugstore in St. Louis, Herbert R. Speckart did not display prices on his vitamin products. He claimed that when prices were shown, customers tended to choose purchases based on cost, sometimes the cheapest, sometimes the most expensive. Speckart preferred that consumers' selections were based on individual need. The pharmacist talked with customers, found out what they wanted, and then explained the merits of various brands, their relative potency, and cost. In this way, price became just another factor in the decision-making process and customers were impressed with Speckart's interest in their problems and his expertise. This, the druggist believed, resulted in many repeat customers.[19] Paul Clark in St. Marys, Kansas, took the personal approach as well, but he did not limit himself to product recommendations. Considering it his duty to educate as well as to sell, he discussed the customers' conditions first and then either directed them to specific vitamins or to a physician, if necessary. Consequently, he wrote, "customers know that buying vitamins in his drug store is not the same thing as buying them in a grocery store or variety store when they are sold indiscriminately by untrained, uninformed clerks whose chief interest is to make a sale."[20]

Thwarted by the courts' unwillingness to set a legal stamp on their professional status in terms of vitamin sales, New Jersey pharmacists joined forces to bring the issue to the public. In Essex County, 150 druggists undertook a concerted drive to make February "Vitamin Month." Their slogan, "Now is the time to vitaminize," was blazoned in headlines and in drugstore windows (Figure 3-4). The druggists intended this campaign to have two results: one was to make the public "vitamin conscious"; the other, to convince the American consumer that vitamins should be purchased in the drugstore. This successful promotion, reported to increase sales in participating stores by 20 percent to 50 percent, was repeated every winter for many years.[21]

Pharmacists all over the country designed displays to promote vitamins and to inspire customer confidence. Stores mounted signs headlined "Know your vitamins" and listing facts about the micronutrients. Charts on vitamins and deficiency diseases were favored window exhibits.[22] The science of vitamins was a popular and evidently effective advertising theme.

Several manufacturers assisted druggists in their struggle with nondrug outlets. Vitamins were high profit items, a fact most

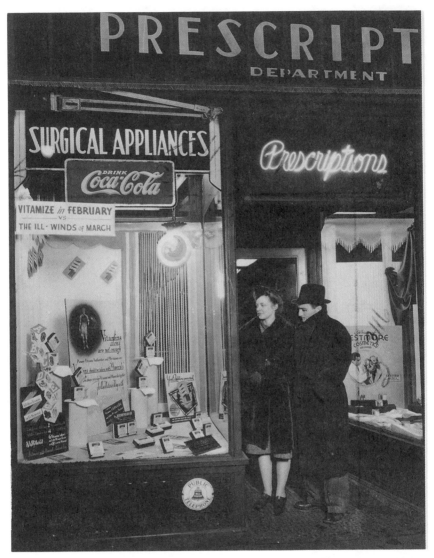

**Figure 3-4:** "Vitamize" window display, Newark, N.J., 17 February 1941. (Source: *Drug Topics* collection. Courtesy of the American Institute for the History of Pharmacy.)

manufacturers stressed in their advertisements to the retail drug trade. Companies provided stores with displays designed to highlight their products and to induce quicker turnover. In addition, national-brand advertising campaigns saved druggists from the expense of devising their own promotions. Typical were Grove's January 1942 double-paged advertisements in the drug trade press that alerted druggists to a "gigantic advertising campaign" consisting of a coast-to-coast radio program on seventy-three stations, every Sunday night; a new coast-to-coast morning radio program on eighty-eight stations, three times a week; and "dramatic, hard-hitting radio spot announcements in 92 cities."[23] International Vitamin Corporation showed its support of pharmacists with the fable of the grocer, the baker, and the vitamin maker. The grocer, the drug-press advertisement warned, was grabbing at the vitamin market because wartime rationing had severely limited sales in the usual lines; the baker was invading the vitamin trade because people believed that buying enriched bread (another emergency war-time measure) provided them with all the vitamins necessary to good health. Nonetheless, druggists who "know their vitamins" can build a profitable department by establishing themselves as "vitamin specialists" and by stocking I.V.C. vitamins, "the vitamin preparations made by specialists."[24]

In addition to this positive support for vitamins in the drugstore, some companies went further and refused to sell their products to nondrug outlets. Those who took this route made sure that pharmacists knew this too. These companies tied their success in vitamin sales directly with that of the drug stores. Grove's advertisements to the retail drug trade repeatedly underscored that druggists needed to "wake up to profits you're losing" to nondrug outlets and reminded them that the widely advertised Grove's Vitamins were "confined *exclusively* to the drug trade! You've got the product—GROVE's Vitamins. Now get the profit!" Other Grove's advertisements were "intended to stimulate awareness among retail druggists of the strong undercurrent of competition in the highly profitable vitamin field. Suggestions offered herein may supply you with ammunition to combat the dangerous upward surge of vitamin sales in unorthodox outlets."[25] Lacking company sales statistics, the success of these specific advertising campaigns cannot be determined. But these examples represent common themes in vitamin manufacturers' advertising to retail druggists.

Whether the advertisements of such national brands directed consumers away from nondrug outlets and into drug stores; or whether the publicity surrounding court cases cued customers to think of vitamins as drugstore items; or whether the promotions of druggists convinced the American public that vitamins were drugstore items; or for some other reason, it is clear that drugstores throughout the decade of the 1940s and beyond continued to dominate the vitamin market, despite pharmacists' frightening predictions. Just as the Kroger/Indiana and other legal cases sputtered out with no dramatic conclusion, so too did the druggists' fight against the grocers. Though pharmacists feared they would lose a significant share of the market to grocery stores, it did not happen in the 1940s. Through the time of the most vitriolic squabbling, drug stores continued to hold indisputable sway.

Vitamin sales consistently increased from the 1920s onward. The earliest year for which we have figures analyzed by place of purchase is 1942, at which time drugstores handled 77.6 percent of retail vitamin sales, including prescription products. Though this share dropped slightly in 1943 to 73.5 percent, it rebounded in 1944 to 77.4 percent and continued to rise each year until the drugstore market share of vitamin purchases reached 87.6 percent in 1948. At the same time grocery sales of vitamins fell from a high of 3.1 percent of market share in 1942 to 1.2 percent in 1947, with a slight rise to 1.3 percent in 1948. Though statistics for other nondrug outlets are less complete for this time period, several did command a greater market share than did grocery stores. For example, mail order houses accounted for 5.1 percent of total vitamin sales in 1947, their share falling to 4.8 percent in 1948. In the available statistics, other outlets such as department stores and industrial sites demonstrate a similar decline through 1948. It is ironic that the outlet that stimulated the greatest fear of competition in the 1940s, the grocery store, played a relatively minor role in nondrug outlet sales.[26]

By the late 1940s, the picture began to change. While vitamin sales remained the most significant category of products on the drugstore shelf, the pharmacy market share began to tumble. Although the figures charted were gathered somewhat differently after 1954, the trend remained consistent. Drug stores were handling a smaller and smaller proportion of the vitamin market. By 1956, only 73 percent of vitamin sales occurred within the pharmacy, down from the high of 87.6 percent in 1948. However, with the rapid growth in the industry as a whole, vitamins remained a bulwark of pharmacy sales, despite the lower market share. In 1948, vitamins had accounted for 4.47 percent of total drugstore sales; in 1956, this figure was only down to 4.02 percent, and it still represented the largest single product category sold in the retail pharmacy.

Given these shifting figures, pharmacists fought even harder to maintain their role in vitamin purchases. In state after state pharmacists turned to the courts and even to legislatures, in a continuing effort to secure legal protection for their particular role in vitamin merchandising. California offers an illustrative case of a battle that extended over more than a decade.

As early as 1942, grocers and other retail merchants petitioned the California Board of Pharmacy to allow them to sell products that were restricted for sale in licensed pharmacies only. Public hearings were held, at which retail druggist organizations such as the Northern California Retail Druggists' Association and the California Pharmaceutical Association argued that such sales were not in the public interest; moreover, they had "not been asked for by the public." A superior court ruling limited the number of drugstore items a grocery could handle. A short time later, the board issued citations to a number of grocery stores in Los Angeles for selling vitamins. This did not end the controversy. Several years later the state legislature considered a bill to license all vitamin sellers. Needless to say, the grocers objected to such licensing. So did the pharmacists who insisted that they should not need another license to sell "anything in the medicinal line."[27] By the early 1950s, evidently California had reached the same level of compromise as many other states, for the Board of Pharmacy found it necessary to remind grocers and other food markets that vitamins with therapeutic claims could be legally sold by registered pharmacists only.[28] By 1953 the state law recognized what had become the commonly accepted division: vitamins taken for the purpose of curing or preventing disease were to be sold only in licensed pharmacies; vitamins taken as dietary supplements could be sold in any store.[29]

California's attorney general (and later governor), Edmund G. Brown, issued a clarifying ruling in 1954 that both strengthened and weakened the pharmacists' position. On the one hand, he sustained the contention that only registered pharmacists could sell vitamins intended for the cure and prevention of disease, though others could sell dietary supplements. On the other hand, he also ruled that a pharmacist could not advertise a vitamin as a specific cure nor diagnose or prescribe a vitamin to a customer. Either activity would be construed as practicing medicine, which a pharmacist could do only as a "licensed practitioner."[30] Pharmacists reacted strongly to this decision, claiming that such a limitation amounted to a denial of their professional obligation. According to Angelo Bosso, a San Francisco pharmacist, professionalism meant using his knowledge and training to inform his customers "concerning the merits, uses, and dosages of such special items as vitamins." Such expertise set druggists apart from grocers and other nonpharmaceutical retailers. Moreover, recommending a vitamin to a customer was not prescribing or practicing medicine, he claimed. If a customer needed a cough medicine and was unable to take codeine, he would suggest a brand without codeine; was this prescribing? If a woman was allergic to certain face powders, was it prescribing to suggest an alternative? Bosso contended that vitamins provided an analogous situation. "If a customer comes in and says, 'I think I need some vitamins,' or 'I have a cold,' or 'I am tired all the time what brand do you recommend?'—have we not a right, in fact, a duty, to tell the customer what we believe is an entirely suitable make of vitamin?"[31]

This predicament, the fine line between the professional duty to advise and the practice of medicine, between the pharmacist

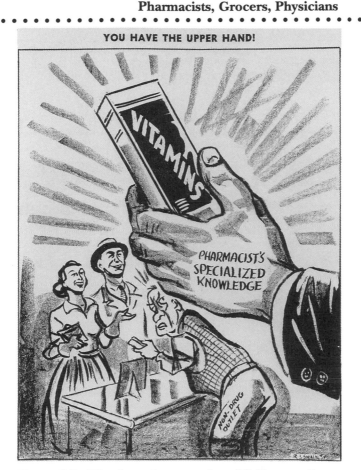

**Figure 3-5:** "You have the upper hand!" (Source: *Drug Topics*, 10 June 1957, p. 44. Reprinted with permission of *Drug Topics*, Medical Economics Publishing, Inc.)

and the physician, did not seem to concern many druggists. They were confident about their activities; they were professionals (Figure 3-5). As the journal *Drug Topics* editorialized in word and picture, it was the pharmacists' specialized knowledge and professional training that set drugstores apart from groceries. Bemoaning the drop in retail druggists' share of the vitamin market in the late 1950s, the editors reminded their readers that unlike vitamin sellers, the retail pharmacist could "place his specialized training and knowledge behind the sale of each vitamin product. Herein lies the drug store's strength. In all probability it accounts

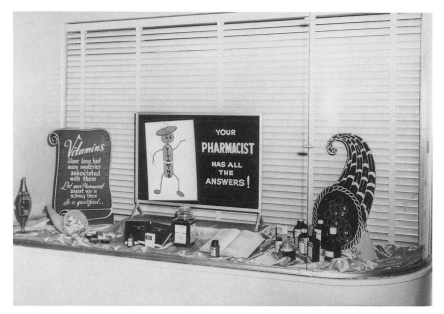

**Figure 3-6:** "You're the expert," 6 February 1967. (Source: *Drug Topics* Collection. Courtesy of the American Institute for the History of Pharmacy.)

for the fact that pharmacies still sell most of the vitamins through-out the country."[32] And it was true that in the late 1950s, cus-tomers preferred to buy their vitamins in drugstores. Since the vitamin market was rapidly expanding, the dollars spent in phar-macies for vitamins increased also.

Though drugstore sales were rising, pharmacies' proportion of the market continued to slip. By 1960 vitamins accounted for only 3.2 percent of the pharmacies's sales, which still, however, repre-sented the largest single product category in the store.[33] In conse-quence, druggists more and more shrilly championed their professional advantage over grocers and other nonpharmaceuti-cal retailers. Judicial and legislative attempts to restrict vitamins to drugstores had both been unsuccessful. Pharmacists focused their attention even more on promoting their professional aura. One sample window display exemplifies this theme (Figure 3-6). The poster on the left declares: "VITAMINS have long had many myste-ries associated with them. Let your Pharmacist assist you in solving them. He is qualified." The center poster reads: "Your pharmacist has all the answers!"[34] As *Drug Topics* reminded its readers, "Nothing impresses the vitamin purchaser more than knowledge of product, and pharmacists with high vitamin sales prove this."[35]

In addition to in-store displays and the "personal touch," media advertising bolstered vitamin sales, and manufacturers aided local pharmacies in attracting consumers' attention. Typical was Squibb's major campaign for its multivitamin product Vigran, whose original announcements publicized the drugstore as vitamin headquarters. The manufacturer described it as "the biggest single-product advertising campaign in the history of the company." Squibb offered druggists a counter display "designed for fast sales action" and promised with it "minimum space—small, compact, under 6 inches square. Maximum profit." Squibb backed this promotion with "big-time advertising" on such popular national television programs as "Mr. Ed," featuring the celebrated talking horse; the popular quiz program "Password"; the renowned mystery series "The Alfred Hitchcock Hour"; and the widely watched CBS news programs featuring Harry Reasoner and Douglas Edwards. The print media was not slighted either. An impressive spread was placed in *Life* magazine, and on the local level Squibb joined with retail drug stores in a cooperative advertising program that included the names of retail pharmacies participating in the plan.[36]

By the mid-1960s, however, the trend was clear; pharmacists' evocation of professionalism was insufficient to stem the tide. Though vitamin sales were increasing across the nation, the drugstore's market share was slowly but steadily declining. Druggists looked back fondly on the golden decade of the 1950s when "members of most American households—including pets—took at least one vitamin pill a day, [and] the drug store was the major outlet for any number of top brand items at full list prices." By 1963 vitamins comprised only 2.3 percent of drug store sales and continued to decline.[37] Over the years increasing numbers of outlets had entered the vitamin market. Now drugstores faced competition from not only grocery stores, department stores, and mail order firms, but also discount drugstores and even door-to-door sales organizations like Fuller Brush. In these troubled times of new markets, salvation lay once again in the professional expertise of the pharmacist. Druggists focused more and more of their attention on special therapeutic formulas, particularly those prescribed by a physician or requested by a customer on the advice of a physician.[38]

But even while pharmacists touted the benefits of their professional advice, the market share for pharmacies dropped to 33 percent by 1981. Though vitamins represented a smaller portion of drugstore sales than in earlier decades, they remained one of the more lucrative product lines. One 1986 marketing survey estimated that vitamin sales averaged $10 a square foot per week, which was better than hair-care and skin-care products and significantly better than overall grocery store sales, which averaged only $8 per square foot per week.[39] Today drugstores continue as the site of one-third of the vitamin sales in this country, amounting to over $1.2 billion.[40]

For many decades, pharmacists had used their professional stature first to claim the privilege to be the sole dispensers of vitamins and then to dispense vitamins for cure, treatment, and prevention. The hard struggle to convince judges and legislators of their right failed. They next turned to the public and sought to convince generally healthy middle-class consumers of the benefits of professional expertise. Temporarily this claim, coupled with the advertisements of national brands that directed consumers to pharmacists, apparently supported the druggists' position in the vitamin market. Clearly, however, the argument of professionalism was not sufficient in light of growing competition. Moreover, the aura of professionalism also lost its appeal. Increasingly, middle-class Americans resisted "received wisdom" and sought their own answers to the prickly question of vitamin supplementation. With the ubiquity of vitamins in American life, combined with the growing self-help movement and the desire on the part of many to take charge of their own health, druggists could not maintain their position in the trade.

Likewise, the self-help movement and the popularity of self-medication provided a ready audience for the claims of Linus

Pauling, a Nobel Prize winner in both chemistry and peace. Furthermore, the scientist's name recognition assured that his opinions, contentious though they were, would be featured in the popular media. The controversy over Linus Pauling's recommended vitamin C therapy threatened a different group.[41] Spokespersons for the medical profession and for nutrition researchers resented Pauling's involvement. They believed that megadoses of vitamin C at minimum were ineffective and a waste of money and at worst dangerous. Likewise, the popularity of a theory proposed by a nonphysician weakened their position of authority in health matters. The altercations between Pauling and his opponents brought the controversial nature of the science of vitamins directly to the American public.

Pauling's advocacy of vitamin C therapy for the prevention and cure of colds threatened the image of science as rational and unambiguous. Over 100 different, easily spread viruses have been causally linked with the so-called common cold. How to judge an individual's exposure to the various causative agents? Some people rarely succumb to colds; others develop many each year. How to control for and evaluate differential susceptibility? How to evaluate the success of any treatment? Lost workdays? A hacking cough? The interpretation of research results and who could interpret them became the central issues in the controversy. Despite vocal opposition from the medical profession, Pauling presented his interpretation with sufficient conviction to persuade a sizable portion of the American population to take vitamin C as a preventive.

Linus Pauling was not the first to consider vitamins a preventive and cure for colds. Popular literature and advertisements linked subclinical vitamin deficiency and respiratory conditions from early in vitamin history. Frequently the evidence was anecdotal,[42] but by the 1930s scientists had begun to investigate the relationship between vitamins and colds. One study gave a group of 185 workers one tablespoon of cod-liver oil each daily; another 128 persons were identified but not given the dietary supplement. Over the course of the experiment, only 44.9 percent of the cod-liver oil group developed colds, in comparison to 67.2 percent of

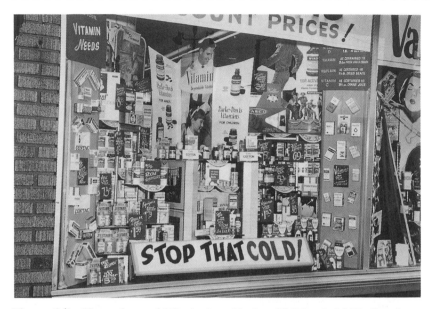

**Figure 3-7:** "Stop that cold!" window display, 29 March 1965. Caption reads: "'Stop that cold!' window sign at Kauffman Pharmacy, Hatboro, Pa., stops traffic cold, and directs their attention to a mass display of remedies. Management notes that the display is 'most effective' in producing sales." (Courtesy of the American Institute for the History of Pharmacy.)

the control group. Moreover, the members of the cod-liver oil group were absent only half as many hours.[43]

Druggists capitalized on consumers' concerns about colds and the availability of vitamin products. Typical was J. A. Reynolds, a Boston pharmacist, who conscientiously courted his customers. Each time a cold remedy was purchased the druggist asked if the patron was susceptible to colds. If the customer answered yes, then Reynolds would explain how customers could use vitamins to fortify against them. Another pharmacist, from Brooklyn, wrote to *Drug Topics* about how he had increased vitamin sales by 25 percent. He simply considered the purchase of a cold remedy "a cue for us to suggest vitamins to help prevent colds in the future."[44] Cold prevention remained a popular vitamin theme among pharmacists (see Figure 3-7).

Within a short time, attention moved to vitamin C. In 1938 in words only slightly less dramatic than Pauling's later declarations, Herman N. Bundesen, a leading midwest physician and president of the Chicago Board of Health, defined vitamin C as the "mystic white crystal of health." He bemoaned the prevalence of vitamin C deficiency in the United States, specifically linking it to "a general run-down condition that makes [people] more subject to colds and other infections."[45] Though he did not advise taking vitamin supplements, he warned that a "good meal" did not necessarily supply all the required vitamins. Mothers, he admonished, must be careful to feed their children orange juice, tomato juice, pineapple juice, or cole slaw regularly. But Bundesen lacked any specific research findings to support this counsel.

As part of the war effort in the 1940s, physicians began to study more closely the effects of vitamins, and of the lack of vitamins, on the human condition. Much of this attention focused on the vitamin-B complex, particularly its influence on the health and well-being of workers and soldiers. Other investigators studied the relationship between vitamin C and colds. The most widely reported experiment in the 1940s took place at the University of Minnesota, where students were given vitamin C pills, multivitamin preparations, or placebos. The result: subjects who received vitamin C experienced fewer colds than previously, but so too did the other two groups. Researchers concluded that for the well-nourished individual vitamin supplementation was ineffective in controlling colds, though they admitted that the case was probably different in situations of malnutrition.[46]

Those opposed to vitamin supplementation were alert to these results. From the earliest days of vitamins, some physicians had always insisted that supplementation was not needed. Leaders of the American Medical Association frequently worked with representatives of the Food and Drug Administration to denounce vitamin therapy as "fraud." They cautioned that little evidence existed to document the power of vitamins, except in clear cases of vitamin deficiency. Physicians dismissed the idea that vitamin supplementation could benefit the cold sufferer. In 1961, *Today's Health*, a popular health magazine produced by the American Medical Association, simply wrote off any connection as "pure superstition."[47]

Though the vitamin-and-cold connection had been debated before the 1970s, the catalyst for the major public controversy was Pauling's *Vitamin C and the Common Cold,* published in 1970.[48] Pauling often repeated the story of his introduction to vitamin C. In 1966, at the age of sixty-five, he attended an awards dinner at which he expressed an interest in living another fifteen or twenty years. A short time later he received correspondence from a member of the audience, biochemist Irwin Stone, who advised that he take daily doses of vitamin C at a level ten times that recommended by the FDA. Pauling and his wife both started following this regime and noticed a feeling of well-being and a decreased number of colds. From these experiences, he postulated that illness could be treated with "substances that normally occur in the body, instead of chemicals derived from plants or synthesized," a practice he termed "orthomolecular medicine." In addition, he hypothesized that the vitamin C needs of individuals vary extensively; some may need 250 milligrams (about ten times the recommended amount in the early 1970s), others may need forty times that.[49] He included these theories and a recommendation that people need massive vitamin C supplements to insure their optimal health in his 1970 publication.

The book was replete with theoretical explanations and Pauling's reanalysis of previous studies. We have no way of judging how much the public read, understood, or considered these sections. But whether or not they cared about Pauling's rationale is not significant. What is important is that they followed his advice. While national statistics are difficult to obtain, the drugstore press often remarked on the upswing in vitamin C sales. Unseasonably cold weather in Florida in December 1970, coupled with newspaper articles quoting Pauling's regime, sent many of the state's residents to their local drugstores for vitamin C. Pharmacists in the Sunshine State reported runs on vitamin C products and calls from customers about the appropriate level of vitamin C to prevent colds. At the northern end of the country, druggists in Minneapolis–St. Paul related similar stories. Consumers were buying up all their stock of vitamin C to prevent colds.[50]

While the public embraced Pauling's claims, the medical profession rejected both his theory and his expertise. Even before the book was officially released, physicians began to assail his authority, criticizing both his scientific explanations and his right to make them. Physicians who opposed him—and they were many and vocal—attacked not only his rationale but also his person. Their resort to *ad hominem* invective weakened their own claims to be objective, dispassionate observers of medical research and undoubtedly attracted even more attention to Pauling and his cause.

And it did become a cause. One of the most frequently cited critics of Pauling's work on vitamin C was Dr. Frederick J. Stare, chair of the nutrition department at Harvard University School of Public Health. A 1969 article in *Mademoiselle* characterized Stare as "one of the country's Big Names in nutrition." After describing the Minnesota research as "a very careful study" that disproved the efficacy of vitamin C in combatting colds, Stare concluded: "[Pauling is] a great man in chemistry and a great American, but he is not an authority on nutrition."[51] Many other reports in the media picked up on this charge. In the same month, *Newsweek* provided readers with a balanced summary of Pauling's book and his advice. It noted that "many [experts] remain unconvinced about claims that [vitamin C] is a remedy for colds" and concluded by quoting Stare that "Linus Pauling is a man of peace and chemistry, not nutrition."[52]

And so the controversy continued over the years. Following the initial publication of *Vitamin C and the Common Cold*, an avalanche of articles publicly debated the use of vitamin C to prevent and cure colds. Whether viewing Pauling as a quack or as a savior, articles in the popular press publicized both sides of the issue. On the one side was Pauling, the two-time Nobel laureate, a man of science who had a cause. "Dr. Pauling" wrote *The Nation*, "is a most responsible scientist. The same concern for human welfare that won him the Nobel Prize for Peace in 1962 motivates this book. He is an outstanding example of the kind of scientist who is more needed now, in an era when the quality of our environment is rapidly deteriorating, than even before—one chiefly concerned with the humanly useful application of scientific knowledge."[53]

On the other side was the medical profession, often with quotations from the American Medical Association or Stare or another named nutritional researcher determined to use professional authority to protect the consumer from, in Stare's words, "false hopes."[54] Opponents did critique Pauling's work. But, as frequently if not more so, they attacked his right to enter into their world; his position as a chemist and a man of peace, they insisted, gave him no license to dispense dietary advice. In their eyes, he lacked the qualifications that would sanction his advocacy of vitamin C.[55]

Critics frequently pointed out that Pauling did not conduct any of the research himself. Moreover, they claimed, the researchers who had conducted the original work concluded that vitamin C had no effect on colds. Thus Pauling was censured for differing with the very scientists who ran the studies and who had more experience and expertise in these areas.[56] In his defense, not surprisingly, Pauling positioned himself as an even better scientist than those too blinded by conventional wisdom to see the benefits of vitamin C therapy. In answer to the charge that his book was based on speculation, not research, he angrily replied: "I didn't 'speculate' about vitamin C. . . . My book is largely a discussion of the published *evidence* about vitamin C in relation to the common cold. The various studies—often double blind studies—carried out by physicians using approved methods have *all* shown with statistical significance—high statistical significance—that 200 milligrams of vitamin C a day has protective effect against the common cold." Why, then, an interviewer asked, is there so much skepticism in the medical profession? Pauling responded that people in medical schools and schools of nutrition denied the efficacy of vitamin C merely out of "habit." He, however, "decided to read *all* the published papers on vitamin C, to examine the data, to repeat the calculations." He quoted nineteen studies in his book that provided "convincing published evidence of the value of vitamin C against the common cold." Nonetheless, he suggested that a more elaborate, closely controlled, long-term project still needed to be conducted.[57]

From their professional position as experts, medical opponents not only denied the possibility that Pauling could analyze and

interpret nutritional data, they implied that laypersons were incapable of evaluating competing claims. Commentators blamed the
increased sales of vitamin C products on a gullible public taken in
by "wild" conjectures and Americans' "historic need for bottled
voodoo."[58] For those with faith in the power of vitamin C, no evidence would dissuade them from taking vitamin supplements. Dr.
Charles Glen King, a member of the team that in 1932 isolated
vitamin C, was very understanding: "Why is it that the average
layman likes to believe that extra doses of vitamins will cure his
ills? I think the answer is fairly obvious. We all like to believe in
miracle drugs."[59] But was it simply faith in a "miracle drug," an
irrational desire for an "easy fix"? Or did the public's overwhelming response to vitamin C therapy involve more? Were consumers
incapable of understanding or uninterested in the scientific evidence? Or, were they evaluating conflicting claims and drawing
their own conclusions?

Clearly, despite the vigorous attacks on Linus Pauling and his
theories, despite the opposition of the AMA, the National Research Council, the FDA, and other prestigious scientific bodies,
there was not unanimity in the medical community. In 1968, the
United States Department of Agriculture had advised the public
to increase the use of oranges, grapefruit, and tangerines as a
preventive against the common cold. The Food and Drug Administration had previously categorized vitamin C as a substance
"Generally Recognized as Safe," but in the early 1970s it was rethinking that classification. The British Medical Association's recommended daily allowance of vitamin C was less than one-third of
the U.S. recommended level.[60] The renown of Pauling crystal-
lized, personalized, and brought to the public's attention differences that existed within the medical community earlier and had
continued unresolved.

The popular media continued to follow vitamin C research. In
a 1972 University of Toronto study, half the subjects were given a
gram (1,000 milligrams) of vitamin C daily, the other half a placebo. The aftermath of this project demonstrated the difficulties
in interpreting such data. Among the subjects in the vitamin
group, one-quarter remained free of colds; among those in the

placebo group, one-fifth did—a difference, but not a statistically significant one. Also, the vitamin group missed one-third fewer work days, perhaps because their colds were milder. There were, however, several problems with the study. Vitamin dosages were not regulated; members of both groups could take additional vitamins, if they wished. No data was collected on previous work histories or on current work situations. Was this data significantly different from the subjects' previous experiences with colds? Were people in particular work settings more likely to stay home than others? Philip White, the director of the AMA's Department of Foods and Nutrition, concluded, "There are just too many subjective factors; valid research in this area is extremely difficult." Yet the author of the study, Dr. Terence W. Anderson, who set out expecting to prove Pauling wrong, ended with the belief that "the intake of additional vitamin C can lead to a reduced burden of 'winter illness.' "[61]

Other studies by the National Institutes of Health, by the University of Maryland, and by the Public Health Service at an Arizona boarding school for Native American children presented similarly ambiguous results.[62] In June 1974, *Changing Times* declared that "thirteen studies made between 1942 and 1974 by investigators other than Pauling indicate that [vitamin C] is virtually worthless in preventing or shortening colds." The next month *U.S. News & World Report* confidently announced to its readers that "recent scientific studies indicate that large intake of vitamin C may, indeed, have this effect." When the *New York Times* reported in 1975 that the *Journal of the American Medical Association* (*JAMA*) had published two reports demonstrating that "vitamin C showed little merit in treatment of the common cold," Pauling felt compelled to respond with a letter to the editor, pointing out the omissions in the studies. This, in turn, elicited a defense of the reports from *JAMA*'s editor. He was, perhaps, shaking his head sadly when he opened his reply with "One cannot help but admire Dr. Pauling's dogged, quixotic crusade on behalf of vitamin C." After explaining the articles, the *JAMA* editor concluded: "Despite the lonely protestations of this distinguished scientist, we must advise the American public that vitamin C remains unproved as an effective agent in the prevention and cure of the common cold."[63]

Though physicians scorned Pauling, the public found reason to believe in his cause. If the debate between pharmacists and grocers sputtered out in the 1960s, that between physicians and Pauling sputtered on. Popular periodicals discussed new studies that purported to demonstrate the effectiveness or lack of efficacy of vitamin C. These would be quickly followed by an article quoting the reverse claim by the opposition. As investigations accumulated, however, more and more articles appeared quoting researchers announcing that they took vitamin C supplements. Given the popularity of vitamin C, many probably agreed with the *Saturday Evening Post*: "Tests from around the world are proving the validity of Nobel laureate Linus Pauling's theory about the prophylactic benefits of vitamin C. . . . Our country should look upon Dr. Pauling as a valuable national resource."[64] Headlines such as "Dr. Pauling Was Right" appeared more frequently and noted in a matter-of-fact manner that vitamin C was "reported to reduce severity of the common cold" and "may lessen the severity of cold symptoms in some people."[65] Journalists noted that people differed in their vitamin C needs, so much so that "smokers, birth-control-pill users and the elderly may require additional C." Some researchers, such as Anderson of Toronto, claimed that most people needed between 100 and 150 milligrams of vitamin C daily (significantly more than the FDA-recommended daily allowance), and as much as 500 milligrams daily when ill.[66] By the late 1980s, vitamin C was the most widely used single-vitamin supplement in the United States. In 1993, the sales of vitamin C supplements reached $430 million. It was taken daily by 35 percent of the population and by 91 percent of those who took supplements regularly.[67]

Many of the same factors that influenced the general acceptance of vitamin supplementation help explain the continuing popularity of vitamin C. Americans tend to self-medicate. Throughout the twentieth century, we have increasingly questioned the healthfulness of the American diet. At the same time, we have expressed a loss of faith with the medical profession.[68] But, it is important to note, there has been no similar loss of faith in science. In the specific case of Pauling and vitamin C therapy for colds, other elements enter the equation. Cold remedies treat only the symptoms of colds, not the cold itself; consumers have a need for a cure. Pauling was twice a Nobel laureate, which made him a credible spokesperson on scientific matters. In reaction to Pauling's widespread media attention, his opponents did more than point out the holes in his scientific and theoretical stance. They made a cause out of Pauling by criticizing him personally. A 1975 article reported Stare's assessment: "Like Hansel and Gretel, this very intelligent, likable man is lost in the woods of health and nutrition, areas outside his competence."[69] These *ad hominem* attacks made opponents look petty. Their position was further undermined by the reams of conflicting data published in the popular press. If physicians, those who put themselves forth as experts, cannot agree, then maybe Pauling, a brilliant scientist, has a point.

Druggists in the 1930s had begun with a relatively simple question: are vitamins to be considered food or drugs? Pharmacists were professionals who knew about drugs; grocers were not. By the time physicians entered the controversy with Pauling, the question has changed. Vitamins were generally available in many retail outlets. It was not an issue of who could sell vitamins, but who could interpret the research, who could judge vitamin supplementation for a generally well-nourished public. Medical practitioners claimed that their training and research, in other words, their profession, gave them the authority. Yet given the stature of Pauling and the contradictory research stories in the press, it was difficult to persuade a wary public that there were unambiguous answers and that physicians alone held them. In the postwar era, pharmacists and physicians sought to maintain the superiority of professionalism at a time when professional authority was increasingly questioned. In the self-help movement, the civil rights movement, the women's movement, and the anti-war movement, Americans were challenging traditional power structures and traditional social roles. This did not lead to rejection of expertise or a denial of the benefits of science; it did lead, however, to a reevaluation of the role of experts.

# CHAPTER 4

• • • • • • • • • • • • • • • • • • • • • • • • •

# Miles One-A-Day
## The History of a Vitamin Dynasty

For both pharmacists and physicians the central question was: who decides? For them the answer lay in the authority of their profession, professionalism based on scientific expertise. The question, though, would not have been raised without the existence of a flourishing vitamin industry. The science of vitamins provided the knowledge that created a profusion of products; it also provided the grist for the advertising mills that promoted the industry. From its inception, the industry reached beyond consideration of gross vitamin deficiency conditions such as rickets and beriberi. The cure and prevention of these rare conditions could not have sustained a multibillion dollar industry in this country. It was the sale of vitamins to apparently well-nourished middle-class consumers that supported the expansion of vitamin manufacture. This segment of the American public had the financial wherewithal to purchase vitamin supplements; they were concerned for their families' health. Commercial firms were and are well aware of the power of scientific rhetoric in American culture. The cultural authority of science sells.

Over the decades scientists and technicians were able to isolate and synthesize the micronutrients more easily and cheaply. Their work was followed by many, many manufacturers racing into the vitamin market. Some of the earliest entrants into the field were the large, so-called ethical pharmaceutical companies such as

Squibb and Parke-Davis. These ethical manufacturers were closely identified with prescription drugs, but were also involved in proprietary, over-the-counter products. Substantial sales resulted from physician prescription or recommendation and thus ethical companies directed much of their advertising to the medical profession. Other companies were associated more with the proprietary medicine business; firms such as Lever Brothers and Miles Laboratories advertised their products directly to the consumer. Many vitamin companies were small firms, composed of a few people producing only a single product or products for regional sale. The promotion of vitamin products reflected a similar range. The ethical firms tended to be somewhat more circumspect in their claims; most of their advertising budget was spent convincing medical practitioners and pharmacists that their products were useful and needed. Proprietary firms, though, concentrated their advertising attention on consumers.[1] Despite their differences, all these companies shared one important characteristic: they used science and scientific argumentation to sell their vitamin products.

Two companies, Miles Laboratories and the Pannett Company (which will be discussed in the following chapter), illustrate different aspects of the emerging vitamin industry. Miles was already a major national proprietary house before entering the vitamin field. Its Alka-Seltzer product had created a commercial stir with its bold claims and creative advertising. It had also attracted the attention of federal regulators. Pannett was very different. It was a small company, created to market one product, Acnotabs. The distinct experiences of these two firms illustrate how the cultural authority of science was used to market and control the marketing of vitamin products in the mid-twentieth century.

The history of Miles Laboratories and its extremely popular line of One-A-Day products is an instructive example of a successful vitamin producer; the firm utilized contemporary science and medicine to create, develop, expand, and defend its markets. In its drive, Miles used current nutritional science to shape the One-A-Day line. Its promotional and educational campaigns that aimed at generally healthy families were based on current nutritional science. In the offices of regulatory authorities, and the halls of Congress and the courts, the company defended its products with current nutritional science.

Miles Laboratories released its first vitamin product, One-A-Day (Brand) A & D, in the fall of 1940.[2] At the time it was one of many such supplements available to American consumers. However, few products exhibited the longevity of Miles One-A-Day. As one company history explains, the continuing prominence of Miles was a result of its commitment to the public and the public's needs:

> Miles, as a pharmaceutical manufacturer, has conscientiously striven to educate the public about vitamins. The company has always been anxious to disassociate itself from the extravagant claims of faddists and to combat a real and continuing ignorance on the part of the public—and to a large extent the medical profession—regarding the complex nature of the relationship between the micronutrients and good health. Miles has always been sensitive to the needs of consumers and responsive to their changing lifestyles, while at the same time remaining proud of its commitment to ethical standards for its products.[3]

This analysis is true, as far as it goes. From the outset of its vitamin promotions, Miles consciously differentiated itself from the more flamboyant claims of other, less prudent manufacturers. Labels and advertising were scrutinized carefully to insure they were in accord with contemporary science. The company did not promise miracle cures, the hallmark of less cautious manufacturers. Instead, it honed in on anxieties about hidden subclinical deficiencies in apparently well-nourished Americans; over and over it drove home the importance of vitamin supplementation as nutritional insurance. In all this, Miles prided itself on maintaining scientific and medical respectability.

But other factors contributed to the One-A-Day's success as well. Miles remained committed to vitamin products, even in the early years when they were not profitable. Creative and expensive forms of advertising, such as nationally distributed booklets and nationwide radio and television spots introduced One-A-Day to a wide consumer market. Advertising was also used to generate interest among pharmacists. And, in contrast to some others in the vitamin industry, Miles did not attack regulators but reached out for their advice. The history of the development and growth of One-A-Day products exemplifies the enlightened self-interest of one manufacturer and documents how one company parlayed a critical reading of contemporary science into support for its product line among middle-class consumers and policy makers.

The driving force behind Miles's dedication to vitamin supplementation was Walter Amos Compton, grandson of one of the three founders of Miles Laboratories.[4] Compton attended Princeton University, earning a degree in chemistry, and then Harvard University Medical School, graduating in 1937. Following an internship at Billings Hospital in Chicago, Compton joined the company in 1938 as medical and research director. According to company lore, Miles's interest in vitamins is directly attributable to his years as a medical student. At Harvard he became fascinated with the relationship of nutrition to health. From the beginning of his long tenure at Miles, Compton called for the company to enter the vitamin market. Once the company agreed to produce a vitamin product, Compton initiated a series of conferences with representatives of the Food and Drug Administration. He used these meetings, which were unusual for vitamin producers, to solicit comments from regulators about One-A-Day cartons and inserts.

Though it was not common, a few manufacturers did sometimes request premarketing sessions with the FDA. The agency could and did seize products it considered mislabeled, either in terms of ingredient lists or claims. The case of Pannett's Acnotabs, discussed in detail in the following chapter, is a clear example of this regulatory procedure. To reduce the chances of such action, some companies sought premarketing discussions to smooth out potential problems before they threatened marketing efforts. But Compton had a more specific reason for concern. Just as he was assuming the position of medical director at Miles, the company faced a serious challenge from another federal regulatory agency, the Federal Trade Commission.[5]

For many years, Miles's sales and advertising had been dominated by one product. Alka-Seltzer was an "effervescent, analgesic, alkalizing tablet" promoted for "nagging, everyday aches and pains—colds, headaches, upset stomach, various minor muscle and rheumatic complaints, painful menstruation, and over-indulgence." In the 1930s, Miles touted Alka-Seltzer as a corrective for "systemic excess acidity," a condition that supposedly caused various physical problems such as colds and other respiratory ailments. The FTC considered this advertising "false, misleading, and deceptive." Company historians relate that Compton was horrified to learn that there was no scientific or medical evidence to support the Alka-Seltzer claims. Miles was forced to drop the notion of systemic acidity and to stipulate that it had no basis in contemporary science. In reaction, Compton declared that henceforth the company would have all its advertising reviewed by licensed physicians.[6] Doubtlessly the Alka-Seltzer encounter, remembered in the company as "The Stipulation," made him sensitive to the power of federal regulatory agencies. It was not unexpected, then, that he deemed it prudent to have the labeling of One-A-Day reviewed by the FDA.

At least as early as 12 August 1940, Compton and an associate, Jack W. Clissold, visited E. M. Nelson, director of the vitamin division of the FDA, and other agency representatives. Compton brought an artist's sketch of the proposed packaging for Miles's first vitamin product, One-A-Day (Brand) Vitamins A & D, and asked for comments. In the detailed discussions that followed, it was clear that the FDA wanted all pertinent information given to the consumer. Wary of false or misleading labels, Nelson took exception to the statement, "Two or three tablets daily will be found to be of value following operations, fractures, and as an important addition to convalescent diets." He insisted that scientific evidence did not substantiate the claim. Compton concurred, accepting that "the statement perhaps implies unwarranted value." He agreed to drop the reference to operations and fractures and to replace it with "a general statement recommending the product as a part of convalescent diets."[7]

This conference, amicable though it seemed, did not end the matter. As Miles developed more extensive packaging, and

especially carton inserts, the company passed them on to the FDA
for its opinion. The agency had no comment on the package for-
mat Miles sent on 2 September, except to remind the company
that the FDA was putting together new regulations for vitamin
products that "may necessitate some label changes when the regulations become effective." Miles "appreciated" the fact that additional labeling might be called for and noted that a company
representative would probably attend the hearings discussing the
new regulations.[8]

The give-and-take between the FDA and Miles continued even
after the product was placed on retail shelves. The company
passed each new version of its packaging and inserts on to the
agency; the FDA dissected each paragraph and sentence in the
material, even those previously accepted. The FDA objected to
broad health claims for One-A-Day, especially claims that suggested the product "can be relied upon to restore or maintain
good health or to be of general value in the treatment of all illnesses." To the agency such pronouncements sounded sus-
piciously like claims for therapeutic agents. George Larrick, the
acting FDA commissioner, reminded Clissold that strict guide-
lines governed the marketing of therapeutic products.[9] Since the
company was marketing One-A-Day as a supplement, not a treatment, Miles intended to avoid these.

The agency challenged many of the scientific claims included
in inserts, worried that they would confuse consumers. Nelson, for
example, objected to this sentence: "Vitamin A is necessary as an
aid in building natural resistance to infections which are more
likely to occur in the membranes of the nose, throat, eyes, ears,
sinuses and upper respiratory tract when there is a deficiency of
this vitamin in the body or diet." This reference, he protested, led
consumers to believe that One-A-Day was "of great importance in
preventing or treating various infections including the common
cold." He did not agree with this, considering that "the qualifica-
tion 'when there is a deficiency of this vitamin in the body or diet,'
does not, in our view, correct the probably misleading connota-
tion . . . because the average individual is not in a position to
determine whether his lack of resistance to infections is due to a

vitamin A deficiency or to the many other causes of such a condition."[10] In this as in so many other examples, the agency saw its role as protecting the uninformed consumer from bewildering and potentially misleading scientific labeling.

One of the paragraphs questioned by the FDA concerned directions for use and spoke explicitly to the image Miles sought to create with consumers. The focus of One-A-Day's promotional campaigns was the vitamin tablet as health "insurance" for those generally healthy: "Don't tuck the bottle away in your medicine cabinet. Don't take the tablets at irregular intervals or only when you are feeling ill. 'One-A-Day' brand Vitamin A and D tablets are food supplements, and should be taken one a day—every day— preferably with a meal. You will not get the greatest benefits from 'ONE-A-DAY' tablets unless you take them regularly."

Nelson objected; as he read it, these statements implied that "vitamins A and D are a treatment for illness."[11] Such implication would define One-A-Day as a therapeutic product, something quite different. Larrick opposed these statements as well, explaining that they were not "in accord with generally accepted scientific opinions."[12] In the FDA's eyes, Miles's claims suggested that even well-nourished consumers risked vitamin deficiencies unless they took One-A-Day everyday. Larrick found this recommendation unacceptable and false. He and numerous other FDA officials consistently maintained that the general American diet contained sufficient sources of all the vitamins needed for a healthy diet. They balked at any suggestion that vitamin supplementation was necessary or that the American diet was insufficient without daily vitamin supplementation. They insisted that Americans could and should get their vitamins from food. Labels suggesting otherwise were simply using the rhetoric of science to delude the American public.

Yet the idea that the American diet was possibly deficient and that therefore the consumer needed the assurance of a daily vitamin tablet was the rationale for vitamin supplementation. Even more significantly, it was the hallmark of the Miles One-A-Day campaign. Consequently, Miles faced the problem of recommending daily vitamin supplementation in a way that the FDA, a group adamantly opposed to vitamin supplementation, would find acceptable. This it did by skillful indirection. The new inserts read: "'One-A-Day' (brand) Vitamins A and D Tablets furnish an easy, inexpensive way to insure that you get enough of these essential Vitamins. Why not put the bottle on the breakfast table as a pleasant reminder to make taking a tablet every day a part of your daily routine?"[13]

Though Miles reworded this and other sections of their labels and inserts, the company did not agree with all the FDA suggestions. It is important to note that the agency did not give a final approval to any of the Miles labels; that was not its view of pre-marketing conferences. The agency would advise companies, but that was all. Once the product was on the market, if the label were deemed false or misleading, then the FDA would act. At least one FDA agent in early 1942 found the claims on One-A-Day "rather extravagant" and questioned what should be done. By this time, Miles had been negotiating with the agency for almost two years, each time voluntarily sending officials its material. The Chicago office noted the considerable discussions already held between the agency and the company and recommended waiting.[14] Though the agency was not completely satisfied with the labels, it apparently did not think the situation serious enough to remove One-A-Day from the market.[15]

While the company was discussing labels with the FDA, it was simultaneously gearing up for a major advertising campaign to introduce One-A-Day A & D to the general public and to pharmacists. Miles had learned valuable lessons from its success with Alka-Seltzer; consequently, it constructed an aggressive promotion using the power of both print and radio to announce the new product. One-A-Day was advertised in popular magazines such as *Good Housekeeping* and *Parents' Magazine,* and it received the *Good Housekeeping* guarantee seal and the *Parents' Magazine* seal of commendation. Advertisements were heard on such popular radio shows as "National Barndance" and "The Quiz Kids."[16] Announcements in the trade press notified pharmacists about the product and about the national radio campaign that would bring customers into the drugstore. By 1946, Miles proudly informed druggists that One-A-Day products appeared on "Quiz Kids" on 138 stations, "Lum 'n' Abner" on 245 stations, "Queen for a Day" on 138 stations, and other nationally aired popular radio shows.[17]

Whether in print, on the radio, or later on television, One-A-Day advertising campaigns in the 1940s and 1950s consistently invoked education, insurance, cost, and product identification. Promotions sought to educate readers and listeners in the science of vitamins and about the importance of vitamin supplementation for their health and the health of their families. Considering the significance of vitamins for all-around good health, advertisements emphasized, consumers needed the insurance of a daily multiple vitamin. Then, advertisements presented One-A-Day as the most cost-effective vitamin supplement. The tag line reminded consumers to "Look for the Big *One* on the Package."

The themes of low price and product identification were, of course, standard elements in advertising, while those of nutritional science and nutritional insurance resonated with discussions in contemporary popular literature. Advice columns and articles typically instructed consumers on vitamins and appropriate food sources, and some even counseled consumers to be extra safe with nutrition "insurance." "There is one way of being on the safe side, however," a *Good Housekeeping* article explained in 1939; "that is to add a sufficiently large factor of safety to the average minimum vitamin requirement to cover possible contingencies. That's the insurance method, and it's being widely practiced in dietetics today." So the advice was to eat vitamin-rich foods and "take your vitamin concentrates."[18]

The Miles's advertisement in *Parents' Magazine* (Figure 4-1) dramatically displayed the motifs of science, insurance, cost, and name recognition.[19] Contrasting old and new methods of child-rearing and reflecting the ideology of scientific motherhood, the 1941 advertisement dismissed "Dear Old Grandma" and her advice as old-fashioned and ignorant. While presenting a dismaying image of the past, the advertisement described a hopeful future: "What men can dream of—Science can do."[20] "Now we know how essential Vitamins are in our everyday life," affirmed the advertisement. With One-A-Day, consumers need not "risk the diseases

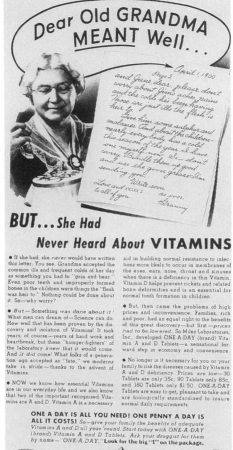

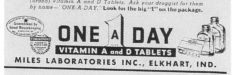

**Figure 4-1:** Miles One-A-Day advertisement. (Source: *Parents' Magazine*, December 1941, p. 80.)

caused by Vitamins A and D deficiency." Only a penny a day could "insure normal daily requirements." Prominently displayed on the bottles and packages and in the advertisements was the big "1." Not just any Vitamin A and D tablet would do, the consumer was told; be certain to get Miles One-A-Day.

One-A-Day Vitamins A & D was not the only product in the line.

By 1942, it was joined by One-A-Day B-complex, which inspired copywriters to poetry:

> The One-A-Day vitamin twins are we,
>     B Complex and A & D,
> And we're the ones, we must confess,
>     Who give you more, yet cost you less.[21]

Miles also stepped up its aggressive advertising, developing a more educationally oriented strategy. In 1942 it produced a sixteen-page booklet to be distributed through drugstores.[22] "Your Vitamins: An Important Subject Explained in Simple Terms the One-A-Day Way" marshaled arguments current in the mainstream press in support of vitamin supplementation. Intended to "cover [the subject] from the scientific viewpoint, but in language not difficult for the general public to grasp," the publication used science as a selling tool. For example, in response to the question "What are vitamins?" the booklet declared: "Vitamins are organic chemical substances found in nature, in small amounts, in foods of animal or plant origin or they may be made (synthetically) in chemical laboratories. . . . Vitamins are chemical substances of vital importance. Without Vitamins life is impossible."[23] "Do we get enough vitamins?" asked the booklet, which then reported on the host of surveys documenting that the average American diet did not furnish the necessary vitamins. Its explanations echoed common concerns found in popular literature: that water-soluble vitamins are discarded with cooking water; that the heat of cooking destroys vitamins; and that modern refining methods strip vitamins from food. In addition, certain conditions, such as pregnancy, illness, and stress, may increase one's need for vitamins. The booklet concluded on an ominous note: "Widespread symptoms of deficiency diseases are seen" throughout the country. "Your Vitamins" went on to describe in detail the conditions that can arise from vitamin deficiencies and to extol the merits of One-A-Day Vitamins A & D and Vitamin B Complex tablets. This bleak picture logically led to the recommendation of a daily vitamin pill to insure the necessary minimum requirement.

Though Miles was marketing products that offered the known

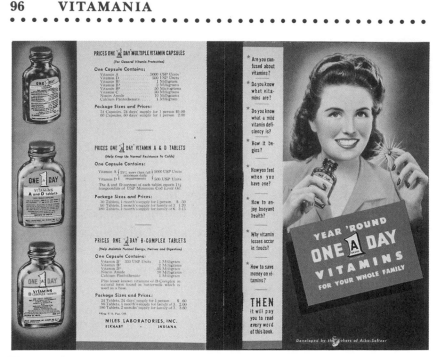

**Figure 4-2:** "Year 'Round: One-A-Day Vitamins for Your Whole Family." (Courtesy of Miles Laboratories Corporate Archives.)

range of vitamins, Compton's original goal had been for a single daily vitamin. By December 1943, despite wartime exigencies and technical difficulties, Miles One-A-Day Multiple Vitamin Tablet was released. Yet, even with three daily vitamin products, throughout most of the 1940s the One-A-Day line was either not profitable or only marginally so.[24]

In an effort to develop a consistent market for One-A-Day products, in 1943, Miles initiated an impressive new campaign, beginning with the publication of "Year 'Round: One-A-Day Vitamins for Your Whole Family." The booklet was flashier than "Your Vitamins," but it dispensed similar information and advice, carefully footnoted to books and medical journal articles written by leading nutritionists and physicians (see Figure 4-2).[25] To draw the reader in, its cover listed common questions about vitamins. "Are you confused about vitamins? Do you know what vitamins are? Do you know what a mild vitamin deficiency is?" The headline on page one informed readers that "millions of Americans are living on diets low in vitamins"; the text warned that three out of four people are "not enjoying the full zest and vigor of robust health largely because they do not eat properly." Vitamin pills are important not just to avoid gross deficiency conditions like pellagra. Consumers who considered themselves healthy should be alert for subclinical deficiencies. This alarm was repeated several times in the booklet, coupled with scary reminders that one cannot always recognize a vitamin deficiency and hopeful reminders that with sufficient vitamins one could "enjoy buoyant health." Citing studies published in the *Journal of the American Medical Association* and the *Archives of Internal Medicine,* "Year 'Round" asserted that in thousands of American households, people were unknowingly experiencing symptoms of vitamin deficiency, including "low resistance to colds, irritability, fatigue, loss of vitality, weakness, nervousness, indigestion, gas, certain skin troubles, sleeplessness." What to do? Readers found the answer in the headline on the next page: "An easy way to prevent or overcome a mild vitamin deficiency is to eat 3 good meals every day and take One-A-Day vitamins." The tablets were "to help replace the vitamins lost in foods due to processing, improper cooking, and so on. They also supply the vitamins needed each day when you don't select the right foods for your meals."

The list of symptoms related to vitamin deficiency was very long and nonspecific. So how do you know if you are suffering from a mild vitamin deficiency? "Year 'Round" offered a simple test. Add more vegetables, fruits, and milk to your diet. In addition, take One-A-Day for thirty to sixty days. If after that time, "you tire less easily, seem stronger, sleep more soundly, are less irritable, and feel better generally," then continue this regimen. However, if you do not feel better, your condition is probably caused by something other than a mild vitamin deficiency. Then the booklet recommended seeing a physician.

"Year 'Round" was a cornerstone in Miles's One-A-Day promotion program. After World War II, thirty million copies were mailed out to consumers, reaching nearly every household in the United States.[26] But the company relied on other forms of advertising as well. Throughout most of the 1940s, radio advertising commanded the largest portion of the Miles One-A-Day promotional budget. In the 1950s, One-A-Day appeared in television advertising, beginning with "Queen for a Day" in 1950. By 1955, more promotional dollars were spent on television than on any other advertising medium.[27]

When One-A-Day entered the field in the early 1940s, it was one of many vitamin supplements offered to American consumers. And it was not even the biggest. In 1944, *Consumers' Research Bulletin* published a two-part article, "The Ubiquitous Vitamin Preparations," which condemned such products. The authors dismissed the idea that scientific evidence demonstrated the existence of mild vitamin deficiencies and the need for supplementation; they blamed the enthusiasm for vitamins on the extravagant news reports of scientific meetings and new discoveries. While rejecting the need for vitamins, except for therapeutic purposes, the authors evaluated nearly fifty brands of multiple vitamins.[28] Interestingly, One-A-Day was not listed.

Miles's advertising had attracted a great deal more attention by 1945, when an article in the *New Republic* blasted One-A-Day along with a series of other vitamin preparations. "The Great Vitamin Scare" scoffed at the Federal Trade Commission's control of advertising and accused vitamin companies of "often using misleading claims based on scientific half-truths and plain untruths."[29] Its leading example was Miles One-A-Day. Though Miles had cautiously discussed its labeling with the FDA, the company was not as careful with its advertising. The content of one particular One-A-Day advertisement with its emphasis on "nutritional insurance" raised the ire of the author. In the ad, a woman revealed that, following the advice of her doctor, she and her family took One-A-Day "to guard against lowered resistance to colds, . . . and a general run-down condition often due to vitamin deficiencies." Sneered the *New Republic* author, "'Help guard against lowered resistance to colds' is the kind of innocuous language the Federal Trade Commission doesn't quarrel with." Yet, the article pointed out, several recent studies demonstrated that no significant benefit resulted from adding vitamins to an already adequate diet.

"The Great Vitamin Scare" discussed other vitamin products in equally damaging terms. The one bright spot in the article was the author's gleeful observation that the "upward curve of vitamin sales is beginning to flatten out." In the mid-1940s, many proprietary vitamin products dropped from the market. In late 1944, Standard Brands withdrew its product line; Lever Brothers withdrew Vimms in early 1946. By that April, Miles Laboratories was the only major proprietary firm still marketing vitamin supplements.[30] The company remained firmly committed to the One-A-Day line. Recalled one executive of Wade Advertising Agency, describing those years at Miles:

> All our concentration then was on the One-A-Day multiple. They had a lot of stick with that product. They believed in it, and I think Walter Compton had alot to do with it. They stuck with it. It wasn't a profitable product for a long time. The competition was fierce, but they outlasted the competition. We had competition from Lever Brothers with a product called Vimms, which they spent millions of dollars on. We had competition from a product that Standard Brands called Stamms. We outlasted—they weren't terribly hard to outlast. You had ethical vitamins from Squibbs, Upjohn and other companies, and of course there are many more companies with the so-called ethical vitamin business, which are theoretically prescription products. However, they are pretty much all over the counter now, even the therapeutic. But the basic idea behind One-A-Day was to add a daily requirement supplement to people's diets that would be helpful in their daily nutrition. For years Miles stuck to that basic premise.[31]

Advertising, consistent advertising, positioned Miles One-A-Day at the top of the market, a position the company fought to keep. Articles such as "The Great Vitamin Scare" insinuated that Miles's advertising was a creation of a copywriter's fertile imagination, while internal company records show the care with which Compton, medical consultants, advertising executives, and other officials from Miles debated the details of advertisements. At one conference, for instance, it was agreed that, since there was no way to present food comparisons without misleading the consumer, food comparisons would not be used. Similarly the statement, "The harder you work or play the greater your need for vitamins," was rejected and replaced with "When you work or play, you need more of certain vitamins that are in this tablet." The conferees agreed that "Vitamins are health protection" was incorrect. Instead, they suggested three possibilities:

1. Vitamins are essential to health.
2. Good health is impossible without enough vitamins.
3. Are you sure you are getting enough vitamins to protect your health?[32]

Miles's executives clearly walked a narrow line between what they deemed acceptable and what were deemed unacceptable scientific claims.

Though many competitors fell out of the market, Miles vitamin sales did not increase dramatically in the late 1940s. Committed to the One-A-Day line, Miles searched for ways to enhance vitamin sales. One major effort involved the National Vitamin Foundation (NVF). In March 1946, Miles Laboratories joined with other vitamin producers, such as Squibb, U.S. Vitamin and Pharmaceutical Corporation, Lederle Laboratories, Eli Lilly, Merck, and Mead Johnson, to form the NVF, an organization designed to finance vitamin research in private laboratories and universities. In turn, the NVF formed the Vitamin Information Bureau, whose primary task was the production of education materials for students, health professionals, and the general public. In 1960, the NVF established a public relations committee. A significant result of this group was the production of a film aimed at increasing the consumers' awareness of vitamins and the need for supplementation. With activities such as these manufacturers reached beyond their product promotions to instruct consumers in the science of vitamins. In one year alone, 1961, the NVF allocated $100,000 for educational programs to promote vitamin supplementation.[33]

For more than a quarter of a century, Miles was the largest corporate contributor to the National Vitamin Foundation, whose pronouncements closely mirrored the company's claims for nutrition insurance, without, of course, specifying any one particular product. "Vitamins and Your Health," a cartoon-studded brochure prepared in 1964, advised readers that a nutritious diet was composed of "enough of the proper foods consistently." However, for many of us, the text asserted, "those three key words: enough, proper, and consistent—are the catch." Fortunately for the reader, promise existed in the form of supplemental vitamins, which many doctors are recommending "simply so that we can be sure . . . we'll 'get our vitamins.' "[34] Using the same title but with a totally revised text, "Vitamins and Your Health" reappeared in 1970, once again insisting that people should get their vitamins from food, but querying: were they? The text mentioned several studies documenting that the diets of many American consumers were insufficient in some or all the necessary micronutrients. To be on the safe side, then, take vitamins: "'Supplemental' vitamins are available as health insurance for people who don't, won't or for some reason can't, stick to a diet that contains the necessary vitamin requirements."[35] Over and over again these brochures and other educational material from the foundation presented the scientific and medical rationale for vitamin supplementation, outlining how the lack of vitamins affect health, describing studies that show many consumers do not get sufficient vitamins, and noting that physicians recommend vitamin capsules if there was any doubt.

This attention to nutritional science dominated Miles's vitamin projects for decades, even when the impetus for a new product developed outside the laboratory.[36] According to Jeff Wade, long-time advertising executive responsible for One-A-Day promotions,

> we used to find ways to find markets; for example, One-A-Day Plus Iron. The vitamin plus iron was an Agency product to begin with, then picked up by Miles. This is because I read a paper by a professor of the University of Iowa, which basically stated that some 80% or better of the females of all ages (it was a campus study at the University of Iowa, but of all ages), lacked iron and there was a definite place for iron supplementation. We made a presentation on that, along with several other types of vitamin products that the Agency thought might be feasible. That was the one the people down here [at Miles] picked up and went to work on.[37]

One-A-Day Plus Iron promotions received the same painstaking analysis as earlier products. Medical consultants particularly ques-

tioned tag lines such as, "To help assure active, good health." It is
true that we all need a certain amount of iron each day, counseled
one medical consultant, and that by consuming One-A-Day Plus,
"you should be assured of having the daily intake of iron that is
needed. However, this does not mean that the person that has a
sufficient amount of iron is assured good health or assured to be
active." He reminded the company that the product was intended
as a supplemental product, not a therapeutic one. Advertising, he
believed, "should be maintained in this category."[38] And the company agreed, directing the advertising agency that "any claim im-
plying a promise of a specific benefit such as increased pep or
energy, improved health, better health, good health, etc. is not
acceptable" and reminding the copywriters that supplemental
products are "intended for use by individuals in normal good
health and as 'nutritional insurance.' "[39]

Long priding itself on the "educational" aspects of its advertising campaign, in 1960 Miles published a *Life* magazine advertisement entitled, "Vitamins and You."[40] Posed as a series of questions
and answers, this advertisement was unabashed in its promotion
of vitamin supplementation. Its third question asked boldly: "Who
should take vitamins?" The answer was decisive: "Everybody
should take vitamins every day to help them feel their best and to
prevent vitamin shortage." The answers to other questions provided the rationale for this unequivocal conclusion: many people
suffer vitamin shortage; foods lose vitamins in cooking; vitamin
deficiency cannot be easily diagnosed; and the other usual arguments for vitamin supplementation.

This is not to say that everyone was comfortable with the pres-
entation of science in Miles advertisements. In the 1960s, general
reviews of vitamin supplementation and the use of science in advertisements began to focus more critical attention on One-A-Day
promotions. One critic's analysis provides an illuminating description of the advertisement in *Life*: "The ad was elaborately
dignified: the type faces used were small, considering the size of
the ad, and not too bold; the brand name was not emphasized;
the tone of the piece was not that of a salesman trying to peddle
his wares but of a public-spirited organization trying to perform a

service by putting the facts about vitamins before the public."[41] It was just this aspect of "science in the public interest" that worried the writer, who pointed out that Federal Trade Commission officials, officers of the American Medical Association, and nutrition experts despaired at the ways such advertisements manipulated scientific evidence. For example, it was true that the United States Department of Agriculture surveys showed that typical American diets were sometimes below the minimum recommended daily intakes of certain vitamins. Yet, the article explained, these minimums were actually two to three times the amount required. Thus deficiencies need not exist even with diets containing less than the stated minimum. The advertisement's claim was seriously misleading. Most irritating about these deceptive statements was that the burden of proof, or disproof, which is not an easy matter, fell to the Federal Trade Commission. "It is one thing to demonstrate that the information on which an advertisement is based does not really prove that it would be a good idea for everyone to take vitamins," contended the *Science* writer. "It is another and far more difficult thing to prove that there is no reason whatsoever for the ordinary person to take vitamins." Clearly Miles and the *Science* author viewed contemporary science quite differently.

In the early years of the 1960s, attacks on vitamin supplementation in general and Miles products specifically appeared increasingly in the press. They worried Compton, by now executive vice president of Miles, who was also disturbed about declining sales.[42] He was determined to differentiate Miles products from "nonsense and unmistakable quackery" and to enhance the scientific respectability of the company.[43] This he did by carefully orchestrating arguments played in advertisements, press releases, congressional hearings, and court cases and by placing the firm and its products within the realm of principled science. Even in private correspondence Compton portrayed promotions of Miles One-A-Day as "a decent job of service."[44] His spirited defense of Miles One-A-Day exemplified his vision of the company's humanitarian spirit.

Two examples demonstrate how Miles used the cloak of scientific and medical respectability to maintain its position in the vitamin field. The first concerns attempts by the FDA to regulate the vitamin market in the mid-twentieth century. Miles was successful in promoting its view of vitamin supplementation in this instance. The second involves advertising for the specialty market for chewable vitamins. In this case the company was forced to retreat. To blunt the negative impact of the defeat, the company reinforced its image of moderation based on science. In these, as in the past, Miles used authority of contemporary science to sustain the marketability and profitability of its One-A-Day products.

Compton readily acknowledged that unscrupulous manufacturers inhabited the vitamin field. However, he saw Miles as an ethical firm and was angry that critics unilaterally condemned all vitamin supplementation. He accused these commentators of misleading consumers, complaining that "the whole program of vitamin supplementation is suffering seriously from this constantly increasing misrepresentation by 'experts' who should and probably do know better." Most important, he was convinced that the very existence of the One-A-Day line was under threat because these critics would continue to attack until the whole industry collapsed. Compton insisted that Miles had to win the "battle," for "we have nothing to lose and everything to gain."[45]

During January 1963, for example, the hearings of the Senate Special Committee on Aging, headed by Senator Patrick V. McNamara, raised the issue of the nutritional status of senior citizens. Some witnesses had used the hearings as a forum for attacking vitamin supplementation. As a first step in the Miles strategy, Compton used a letter to McNamara to get a statement of the company's position on the record. His letter, and subsequent testimony, laid out significant themes that would be heard over and over again. While endorsing

the exposure and the publicity you have been able to give to proved medical hoaxes, I note, however, in the interpretation in the press a lack of differentiation between the exposure of the charlatan and these areas where there is an honest difference of opinion, even among professional experts, particularly as to the need for vitamins to supplement those taken through the food each of us ordinarily consumes. . . . It concerns me personally both as a citizen and a doctor of medicine and as an official of a firm that is recommending and distributing multiple vitamin tablets to the public.[46]

His letter went on to separate Miles products, important in normal nutrition, from "a various multitude of products, which attempt to hang on the magic of the word vitamin all varieties of spurious and imaginary benefits." He agreed that vitamins "are neither a cure-all nor any form of magic pep pill," yet, he explained, products such as One-A-Day serve the public. His letter contained the same explanations hyped in Miles advertisements and repeated in the publications of the NVF. Compton's statement and variants of it were distributed to members of the committee, other members of Congress, the press, science news writers, various retail and wholesale trade associations, medical journal editors, and the drug trade press, in the awareness that "we have at stake Miles Products' 20-million dollar volume on vitamins."[47]

In its public promotions, too, Miles was careful to dissociate its products from the "quackish" wing of the industry. While instructing consumers about the need for vitamins, advertisements typically reminded readers that One-A-Day products were intended for supplementation. Vitamins were important for good nutrition, but they were not "'pep' pills or magic 'cure-alls' for various illness." One-A-Day tablets were not magic potions, and they should not be used therapeutically; instead, they were a sensible way "to be *sure* of getting enough vitamins."[48]

To further substantiate their scientific credibility, in 1969 Miles funded a study that correlated the findings of seventy nutritional studies carried out between 1950 and 1968. This literature review was published in the *Journal of Nutrition Education*, and Miles distributed thousands of reprints.[49] The company also produced a pamphlet, "Vitamins, Minerals and Americans," consisting of "highlights" from the review article and quotations from leading nutritionists commending the publication.[50] Moreover, as FDA vitamin hearings continued into the early 1970s, Miles sponsored the appearances of nutritionists and physicians who testified to the value of dietary supplements.[51]

Miles executives promoted the scientific basis of vitamin supplementation in the media and in congressional hearings whenever appropriate. For example, Compton appeared before the Senate Select Committee on Nutrition and Human Needs in February 1971. In addition to championing daily vitamins for the general consumer, Compton, now president and chief executive officer of Miles, advocated vitamin supplements in the school lunch program. This suggestion was repeated at the December committee hearings. Miles proudly discussed pilot programs it had sponsored, but the federal government did not follow through on the company's recommendations.[52]

The most direct threat to the marketing of vitamin products occurred in June 1966 with the issuance of FDA proposals on vitamin regulation. The agency rules mandated that all multivitamin products carry a crepe label that read as follows: "Vitamins and minerals are supplied in abundant amounts by the foods we eat. The Food and Nutrition Board of the National Research Council recommends that dietary needs be satisfied by foods. Except for persons with special medical needs, there is no scientific basis for recommending routine use of dietary supplements." Miles was one of the first companies to respond publicly to the FDA's action. In a press release that was widely quoted, the company rejected the agency's claim that there was no scientific basis for daily vitamin supplementation. Defending its history and its position in the field, the company remained "convinced that there is an indisputable rationale supporting the routine use of these products by the general public."[53] Despite the threat of the crepe label, some Miles executives answered with satire. One suggested that a government concerned about informing and protecting the consumer should insist that foods such as lettuce, spinach, canned carrots, and peppers be forced to carry a label stating, "This product contains no significant quantity of nutrients other than vitamins and minerals. Unless your physician directs you need this bulk in your diet, it is recommended that a vitamin-mineral supplement tablet will supply an adequate intake of vitamins and minerals at substantially less cost."[54] Humor, however, could not defeat the FDA's proposals. As will be discussed in chapter 6, Miles and other vitamin manufacturers quickly filed objections, instituted law suits, and were able to deflect the agency from the crepe label.

In essence the FDA could not garner sufficient scientific and medical support for its blanket condemnation of vitamin supplementation. Notwithstanding the FDA's and the AMA's conviction that Americans were generally healthy and got all the vitamins they needed in their diets, others were less sure. Over the next decade the agency significantly modified its stand on vitamin regulation. By 1973, Miles had little to quarrel with the agency's latest proposal. The FDA would permit the unrestricted sale of specific standardized vitamin formulae. The composition of One-A-Day products closely matched these. Consequently, the company reversed its stand on vitamin regulation, commending the FDA regulations as a "responsible exercise of administrative authority which is very much in the public interest."[55] In effect, the FDA regulations mirrored the long-standing differentiation that Miles had sought to make; they allowed the company to separate One-A-Day products from "quack" products.

Miles's strategy had succeeded; it had effectively distanced itself from the quackish wing of the vitamin industry and established its respectability. It did not make outlandish claims for its products; it reflected a more moderate view of nutritional science. The company used that same respectability to disengage from a practice that was increasingly being attacked: advertising on children's television. Chocks multiple vitamins, the first children's chewable vitamins, were test-marketed in 1959 and released nationally in 1960. They were joined a decade later by the Flintstones, and in 1971 by Bugs Bunny Children's Vitamins. In the early 1970s, with these three products Miles Laboratories dominated the field of children's vitamins. In March 1971, the New York City Department of Consumer Affairs questioned the contents of a Flintstones print advertisement appearing in the October 1970 issue of *Good Housekeeping*. The company sent a five-page letter in response, citing publication after publication supporting the

formula of Flintstones and children's need for a daily vitamin supplement. Its reaction was somewhat different when challenged
about television advertising.

One report estimated that advertising on television by Miles
and other vitamin producers amounted to $4.7 million in 1971, of
which $4 million was spent on children's shows. In this era, how-
ever, consumers organizations, such as Action for Children's Television, began calling for control of advertising on these programs.
The Federal Trade Commission held extensive hearings at which
vitamin advertisements on children's programs were singled out
for criticism. Though originally defensive, Miles slowly came to
accept that its position was untenable. In an interesting move, the
company used its image of respectability to justify its withdrawal
from children's television. In a letter to Action for Children's
Television, Robert Wallace, a Miles vice president, laid out the
company's rationale: "We have become increasingly convinced
that continued advertising of our children's vitamin supplement
products in the present type of environment of children's television programs has become no longer in our interest: this relates
especially to some of the highly questionable programming as well
as the number and nature of commercials presently being aired in
the Saturday morning period."[56] The company did not, of course,
say that its commercials were false, deceptive, or lacking a scientific
basis. Rather, it separated itself from "questionable" programming,
just as it had set itself apart from questionable vitamin products.

Over the decades, Miles astutely exploited scientific authority
to gain respectability, a respectability with which the company
developed a highly successful and profitable vitamin line. One-A-
Day products were not intended to treat gross vitamin deficiencies;
instead they were intended for generally well-fed middle-class
Americans concerned about hidden, subclinical deficiencies. The
company's promotional schemes used scientific rationale and
reached out through the print media, radio, television, and direct
mail. In its success, Miles both built on and expanded the demand for vitamin products; it also incited resistance. In the ensuing controversy, critics and supporters alike claimed that science
was on their side.

# CHAPTER 5

• • • • • • • • • • • • • • • • • • • • • • •

# Acnotabs

## Scientific Evidence in the Marketplace

Scientific evidence: necessary but not sufficient for a successful vitamin product. Compton's astute use of contemporary science enabled Miles to build a profitable vitamin industry. But the counterexample of Pannett's Acnotabs shows that scientific claims did not guarantee victory. Companies whose science was farther from the mainstream, whose scientific justification was not in tune with contemporary interpretations, those on the quackish wing of the vitamin industry, suffered a different fate.

While Miles was solidifying its position in the market, numerous other firms introduced new products into the vitamin field. These companies varied tremendously. Some were very large; others were very small. Some, like Miles, prospered selling vitamin products; others were short-lived. Some marketed a range of different products, with vitamins being only one of their interests; others produced only vitamins; some only one product. Pannett Company contrasts dramatically with Miles Laboratories. In many characteristics, Pannett was the converse of Miles. Pannett was very small. It was created and developed to market a single product, Acnotabs. One-A-Day was designed for general use as nutrition "insurance"; Acnotabs was created to treat a specific condition, acne. Despite these critical differences, the companies also shared several very important traits. They both advertised in print and over the air and, most significantly, they both employed scientific and medical arguments to attract consumers and to fend off federal regulators. Miles mounted convincing campaigns that bolstered its sales and kept federal regulations at bay; Pannett was not successful. The demise of Acnotabs proves that the rhetoric of science was not enough to flourish in the marketplace. It reveals that the power of scientific rhetoric has limitations.

Acne, though not life-threatening, mortifies many young people, both boys and girls.[1] Acnotabs' radio advertisements played on the embarrassment and misery that adolescents feel about acne.

> Want to clear up pimples *fast—without* giving up sweets—*without* using messy ointments? That's today's news for every teenager who's been *embarrassed* by pimples week after week—but couldn't find real *help!* It's a revolutionary new *tablet* called ACNOTABS. So why mess up your face with ointments or lotions? Why torture yourself, trying to give up candy, desserts, soft drinks? Instead, *stop* pimples where they *start—inside your body*—with the new *internal* medication, ACNOTABS![2]

Print media advertisements, labels, packaging, and in-store displays made dramatic claims:

> These wonder tablets clear up pimples *from inside the body*—quickly, safely, and even in stubborn cases. ACNOTABS do this by magically providing the nutritional elements you may lack.

The magic may be temporary; even with Acnotabs acne might return, warned the promotions. But recurrent acne could be defeated once again—with Acnotabs.

> Even after ACNOTABS have successfully cleared up pimples, these blemishes may return within a few weeks—but usually in much milder form. In these rare cases, start taking ACNOTABS again, but just one tablet daily should then be all you need, to keep your skin healthy and clear.

Consumers were assured that these words were not mere dreams spun by copywriters; they were based on up-to-date scientific and medical discoveries.

CLINICAL STUDY PROVES AMAZING RESULTS: New ACNOTABS tablets have been carefully and thoroughly tested by doctors. . . . Results were literally amazing.

Acnotabs, advertisements proclaimed, represented "A Revolutionary New MEDICAL PRINCIPLE."[3]

"New medical principle"? "Carefully and thoroughly tested by doctors"? These statements created a regulatory and judicial dilemma. Though products frequently invoked scientific and medical authority in their promotions, the sources for analyzing consumers' decisions and for assessing how the public evaluated scientific claims are indirect at best. We can know that many bought a product, or did not buy a product, but not necessarily why. The case of Acnotabs, however, gives us insight into the quandary of a layperson who must decide between conflicting assertions all presented as scientific and medical expertise. With Acnotabs we can see how people outside the scientific community approached such claims.

In order to pull an item from the market, in the early 1960s the Food and Drug Administration had to prove that a product's label was false or misleading. Following such an FDA seizure, a manufacturer had to go to court and persuade a judge otherwise. The FDA questioned the scientific basis for Acnotabs' claims, forcing Pannett to defend its science. From the Acnotabs case we can analyze how a layperson judged scientific argumentation in advertising.

Even before the FDA entered the scene, Acnotabs' advertising claims had been questioned. The National Better Business Bureau had asked that Pannett substantiate the claims for Acnotabs, a request the company's officers declined. They contended that such information involved trade secrets. But they did offer to make such data available after a patent had been obtained. The NBBB had asked the Federal Trade Commission about the legitimacy of the Acnotabs promotions[4] and had even queried the FDA about Acnotabs' claims. Consumers, meanwhile, had complained directly to the FDA.[5] These actions had little effect.

The earliest record of FDA interest in Acnotabs is an inspection report from February 1960, when an agency employee noted that

• • • • • • • • • • • • • • • • • • • • • • • • • • • • • • • • • • • • •

Jewels Pharmaceuticals of Mt. Vernon, New York, was repackaging a new product for Pannett Company to distribute on the west coast. The inspector felt that the product was an inadequate treatment for acne, though he did not explain his reasons, and urged the agency to consider a seizure. The FDA hesitated, however, worried that if Pannett contested the seizure, the agency would be forced to present clinical evidence of inadequacy, evidence it did not have.[6] FDA officials decided to wait to see if the product became a major seller before pursuing more direct action.

By 1961, the FDA decided to intervene. It seized Acnotabs, using its power to pull products whose labels were false or misleading in any way. Pannett contested the seizure. And so began a complicated story of claims and counterclaims, of expert witnesses contradicting expert witnesses, in which a layperson—a judge—had to decide between competing views of science.

In many respects, the FDA's action in regards to Pannett and Acnotabs was typical of the agency's long-standing interest in vitamin products. The initial 1906 Food and Drug Act might be called the "truth in labeling" act. Labels were required to tell the truth about certain named ingredients; a product containing alcohol or opium, for example, had to be so labeled. About other ingredients, the law simply said that the label could not lie: they could be present but not listed; if listed, they must be present. The legislation was intended to identify products for consumers—in other words, to allow informed consumers to self-medicate. Furthermore, the FDA carried the burden of proof when issuing a charge of mislabeling. In the early years of the agency, the majority of FDA vitamin cases attacked products whose contents lists did not agree with the government's analysis of the product. In addition, as early as 1916, the agency undertook research into the physiological action of vitamins. In 1925, a pamphlet was prepared for consumers who were asking for information about vitamins. Two years later, the FDA conducted an extensive survey of cod-liver oil products and discovered that many labels were not truthful about the product's vitamin content or therapeutic value. Investigations of vitamins expanded in the mid-1930s with the establishment of a separate vitamin division. As more rapid, less expensive, and less cumbersome assay methods were developed, the FDA stepped up the number of products it analyzed. By 1944 about one-third of the products seized for false and misleading therapeutic claims were tonics and other items containing vitamins and minerals. Frequently in such cases, the agency would seize a mislabeled product and the manufacturer or distributor did not even bother to appear in court; it was easier to let the court issue a condemnation order by default.[7]

The 1938 Food, Drug and Cosmetics Act added safety to the agency's legislated concerns. Under the law, manufacturers of new drugs were required to submit an application to the FDA, an application that described the contents, manufacture, and uses of the product and that demonstrated its safety when used according to recommendations on the label. No longer, it appeared, did consumers have, nor could they be given, enough information to evaluate the potential hazards of a new product. The agency was to act as a gatekeeper to prevent the marketing of dangerous drugs. The 1938 act directed that producers provide evidence of safety and ordered that the FDA establish criteria for judging the submitted evidence. Congress had considered legislating a board of scientific experts to advise the FDA on standards of evaluation. Because of disagreements over the membership of such a board, though, the law instead ordered that the agency use "all methods reasonably applicable" to design the necessary standards. Even as early as 1938, the FDA viewed controlled clinical trials as basic to therapeutic research. Reflecting the evolving norms of the research community and the FDA, clinical trials conducted by qualified investigators and with sufficient controls and numbers of cases were rapidly becoming the standard for judging the efficacy of products.[8] The growing attention to clinical trials, indicative of contemporary scientific practice and opinion, would be pivotal in the Pannett case.

The FDA's concern for therapeutic efficacy, however, rarely extended to vitamin products in the 1940s and 1950s; at this time the agency's vitamin cases concentrated on unsubstantiated claims. As in the earlier period, these vitamin seizure cases were infrequently contested or were decided by consent degree.[9] To

••••••••••••••••••••••••••••••••••••••••••••••

avoid possibly sticky questions later, some manufacturers, such as Miles Laboratories, asked the agency to review labels and packaging material before the companies released a new product on the market; although the FDA would not give definitive prerelease opinions, early reviews lessened the likelihood of future legal difficulties. Pannett Company, however, did not consult the FDA about labels before marketing Acnotabs.[10] Neither did it quietly accept the FDA's 1961 seizure.

The FDA made its first seizure of Acnotabs on 12 June 1961. After a series of written interrogatories and responses, the case went to trial in the summer of 1962.[11] According to court testimony, Acnotabs originated in 1954 with Russell D'Argente, a pharmacist from West Newton, Massachusetts. One of his customers was taking a drug compounded of vitamin A and several other ingredients for gastritis.[12] While the record does not say how the gastritis progressed, D'Argente reported that he noticed that the customer's pimples "seemed to get better." The pharmacist then consulted a chemist named Dr. Tracy and consequently prepared a batch of tablets with the ingredients of what became Acnotabs. For four or five months, the pharmacist distributed the tablets to schoolchildren. He then contacted Dr. Theodore Shane, president of Chemix Corporation, who later gave the tablets to some other children. About half a year later, D'Argente approached Pannett president William Morrison about developing the product. Throughout this entire period, the pharmacist never consulted a dermatologist, because he believed that a specialist "would not have been interested since such a drug would hurt his business."[13]

In court testimony Shane testified that he had given Acnotabs to twenty-six patients between November 1957 and April 1961. Some were treated for only six weeks, but others for up to ten months. Shane never established any controls nor gave any placebos. He admitted that he knew little about double-blind testing, except that it was to prevent error. Shane was convinced that Acnotabs was effective against acne, though he was unable to answer many questions about the etiology of acne and its diagnosis.[14]

During the trial, government lawyers developed another interesting point: D'Argente himself was associated with Chemix Corporation, which had been founded in 1954 to develop new products. D'Argente held 10 percent of the Company's stock and was assistant vice president. Pannett paid Chemix royalties for the use of Acnotabs. As president of Chemix Corporation, Shane stated that the company received its first royalty check from Pannett in 1960 and that up to 1962 had received something less than $50,000.[15]

Another witness at the court hearing was William Morrison. He testified that Shane's uncontrolled "study" of twenty-six patients provided the basis for the advertising claim that doctors had tested Acnotabs for more than four and a half months. Another later "study" was conducted by Dr. Joseph J. Kelter, a internist in private practice, who also appeared as a witness.[16]

In 1959, Kelter conducted an informal test of Acnotabs at the request of Morrison. This survey consisted of treating six to nine patients for six to eight weeks; Kelter considered this a clinical study because "when you give pills to a patient, that is a clinical test." He was pleased with the results and so informed Morrison, but Kelter did not use Acnotabs in his practice until September 1961, when he undertook a more extensive clinical study. At this time he enthusiastically distributed the product to thirty-nine patients, telling them that it was a new preparation, a very worthwhile preparation. He did not conduct a double-blind study; he did not believe in using placebos. For evidence of effectiveness, Kelter relied heavily on the patients' own assessments of improvement. Furthermore, in contradiction to Pannett's claim that patients needed nothing other than Acnotabs to treat their acne, Kelter's patients received concurrent therapy, including dietary restrictions, lotions, and steaming, all standard contemporary treatments for acne. Also in contradiction to Pannett's claims, Kelter had no acne patients who were cured after only one bottle (seventy-two tablets) of Acnotabs.

Kelter's testimony aptly outlined the claimant's version of clinical trials and scientific claims: a physician distributed the drug to likely patients and observed the results. Kelter admitted that acne was a condition that "waxes and wanes," that categories of severity and improvement were subjective, and that a primary purpose of double-blind testing was to avoid possible prejudice on the part of the participants. Yet he established no control group. The reason he did not use placebos was because he believed "it would be immoral to give a patient a sugar pill."[17] Kelter's philosophy mirrored that of many physicians at that time. Medical practitioners who resisted randomized clinical trials asked for little proof before adopting treatments promoted as effective. These physicians claimed that it was unethical to withhold potentially efficacious drugs from their patients. Researchers, however, claimed that it was unethical to employ products that had not been adequately evaluated; to them, the routine use of insufficiently tested products was equivalent to clinicians conducting flawed experiments.[18]

In the Pannett case, the government placed on the stand expert witnesses of its own who presented an alternative, more orthodox description of scientific testing. These physicians had not conducted any clinical trials of Acnotabs, a fact emphasized by Pannett's lawyers; instead, they spoke from their experience and the experience of others in the field of dermatology. Both physicians testifying for the government had impressive credentials: Dr. Rudolf L. Baer was at the time professor and chair of the Department of Dermatology at New York University School of Medicine, head of dermatology at Bellevue Hospital, and editor-in-chief of the *Yearbook of Dermatology*, among other positions. Dr. John McCarthy was a board-certified dermatologist with particular experience in treating acne. Baer and McCarthy testified to the complexity and variability of acne. They explained that there were several varieties of acne. Its etiology was unclear but differed among the varieties. Furthermore, there was no consensus on treatment for the various conditions, and in any case therapeutic efficacy differed among patients. The most critical point they raised in their testimony was that acne was a cyclical condition with frequent spontaneous remissions. For these reasons, the doctors emphasized, laypersons would have difficulty differentiating between the various forms of acne and therefore would have difficulty selecting the appropriate treatment in individual cases.

Speaking from their positions as specialists in dermatology, the government witnesses claimed that not all physicians had the medical training and experience to evaluate acne cases. Vitamin A was sometimes used as an adjunct therapy in the treatment of acne, they admitted, but in massive doses, more than found in Acnotabs. In particular the government witnesses stressed the necessity for double-blind testing with a disease such as acne, "which has a course of spontaneous remission and exacerbations, in order to determine that just such spontaneous change is not confused with the effect of the drug."[19]

In the above scenario, the case is fairly clear-cut. To withdraw a product from the market, the government had to prove that the label was false or misleading, and the agency documented at least four such instances. First, there is no one single cause of acne. Second, the product had not been thoroughly tested. Third, even Pannett's physicians admitted that patients did not achieve a cure after only one bottle. Fourth, and most important for the researchers, the consensus of the literature denied the effectiveness of vitamin A treatment in cases of acne. In short, the Pannett Company did not have the evidence to support its claims; its labels were false.

Significantly, both sides emphasized the scientific bases for their opinions. The government presented a relatively unambiguous view of scientific research and its cumulative and communal nature. The work of one research program or an individual researcher is not sufficient to demonstrate the validity of a medical therapy. Quoting from an earlier court ruling, the government affirmed that

> medical science is a mass of transmitted and collated data from numerous quarters; the generalizations which are the result of one man's personal observation exclusively are the least acceptable of all. The law must recognize the methods of medical science. . . . It is enough for a physician, testifying to a medical fact, that he is by training and occupation a physician; whether his source of information for that particular fact is in part or entirely the hearsay of his fellow-practitioners and investigators, is immaterial.[20]

Furthermore, the government contended, results must be explained with commonly accepted scientific theories. The extant medical literature did not support and in some instances even contradicted the claim that an internal vitamin A preparation with the ingredients found in Acnotabs could affect an acne sufferer; therefore, the product was not a cure for acne. For the government witnesses, it was not necessary to actually test Acnotabs in order to make this statement. A knowledgeable researcher who analyzed the extant literature would be certain that the product was not a treatment for acne.

Supporters of Acnotabs defined the scientific enterprise in very different terms. They stressed the positive necessity for testing a therapy. Insisting that one could not be sure of the efficacy of a treatment without a study, Kelter even pointedly stated that "one can never know the value of a drug unless one tests it."[21] The internist went on to assert that having observed the benefits of Acnotabs in his practice, he concluded that its *combination* of ingredients seemed to have some potential for the treatment of acne, regardless of the claims in the medical literature. Thus, to Kelter and other witnesses for Pannett, observation was the test; theoretical explanations could follow later.

Moreover, representatives of Pannett pointed to a major inconsistency in the government's argument. Baer and McCarthy concluded that the available literature provided ample evidence for the ineffectiveness of Acnotabs. Yet the government had planned to conduct its own clinical study of Acnotabs. This fact suggested that the FDA was less than certain about its conclusions and needed a controlled, double-blind trial to prove its point. In response, the government explained that it did not have "any doubts about its position," but that the proposed study was "as a trial tactic which Government counsel request[ed]."[22]

How did the judge choose between these significant differences in interpretation and claims? Which was the more convincing view of science: controlled test and professional consensus or empirical evidence? Ultimately he appreciated both. He agreed with both the government's case against Acnotabs and Pannett's claims for the value of its product:

> As the record stands, the Court has before it the testimony of two well-qualified dermatologists . . . who base the medical opinions expressed upon extensive experience in diagnosis and treatment of skin disease, and their knowledge of medical literature relating to the evaluation of the ingredients of Acnotabs, particularly the efficacy of the vitamin content, for treatment of acne. On the other side, there is testimony of one general practitioner and of a well-qualified internist who treated patients suffering from acne with Acnotabs and observed beneficial results as a consequence of which each expressed the opinion that the drug was effective in substantial degree despite some variations in the extent of improvement among the patients treated.[23]

The judge was most especially impressed with the testimony of Baer and Kelter, though they presented dramatically different conclusions. The FDA clearly gave different weights to the evidence offered by these two, but the jurist did not differentiate between the testimony of an academic researcher and an internist. In the court's opinion, Baer was a careful, if not rigid, researcher, who believed that scientific "findings must be rejected to [sic] toto unless they are the product of the maximum objectivity that can be achieved according to recognized scientific methods of study and test." Baer was a credible witness. The judge's characterization of Kelter was less harsh. He understood Kelter's stand as "taking the position that, when a physician treats a patient and observes results, such results cannot be ignored then though there is no rationale in scientific medical theory to account for them."[24] Kelter, too, was a credible witness. Not that the judge accepted the evidence of Kelter's patients as proving the effectiveness of Acnotabs. Rather he believed that neither side had unequivocally demonstrated Acnotabs' efficacy or lack of efficacy. In his opinion, "it does not seem to the Court that the results of these [Kelter's] clinical studies can be translated into representations that Acnotabs will cure acne or would constitute an adequate effective treatment for the disease." The tests were "not extensive in scope or conducted with controls to assure maximum objectivity in evaluation of result[s]." Yet he was persuaded by the testimony that the drug had some beneficial effects, and, therefore, "it may be that more objective and intensive clinical testing will demonstrate the effectiveness of the drug as a treatment for acne, or the lack of it, in a degree that cannot be determined by the evidence now before the Court."[25] The judge's decision sought to find a middle ground between the demands of orthodox science and the promise of empirical practice. Objective clinical trials were required to evaluate therapeutic efficacy, but the judge would not dismiss the experience of an individual physician.

The presented evidence clearly demonstrated that Acnotabs had been labeled as thoroughly tested and an effective remedy tantamount to a cure. The evidence also clearly demonstrated that the company could not substantiate these claims. Therefore, the product was undeniably mislabeled. Typically in such cases, the court would order destruction of the product. In other words, the judge would wholeheartedly accept the FDA's view. With Acnotabs, however, the judge also accepted significant elements of the company's claims. Rather than denying the efficacy of Acnotabs, he ruled that the product had not been thoroughly tested. He directed that the item be returned to Pannett Company, who then had to redesign the labels in accordance with the evidence.

Pannett Company submitted several alternative labels to the FDA for its approval. Despite the judge's evident support, the company could never construct a label that satisfied the FDA, legally the ultimate arbiter on the labeling of drug products. Statements such as "Acnotabs, an internal preparation beneficial in the treatment of some cases of acne pimples" were unacceptable because they would mislead consumers. All buyers would think that their cases would respond, which was clearly not correct even using Kelter's most optimistic results.[26] Wrangling between Pannett Company and the FDA continued for the next several years with no mutually agreeable labels being devised. When Pannett Company was forced to design labels acceptable to the FDA—in other words, in conformity with accepted orthodox science—the distributor was bound to fail. The product neither fit generally accepted scientific beliefs nor produced unequivocal results; therefore, it was marginalized by orthodox science, which, as expressed by the FDA, prohibited Pannett from marketing Ac-

notabs. The company attempted to go ahead and market Acnotabs with labels it considered acceptable. The government
claimed that the relabeled product was a new drug, thus subject to
current regulations. By this time, 1966, the 1938 act had been
revised with the passage of the Kefauver-Harris Amendment, legislation that significantly strengthened the agency's control over
the marketing of new drugs and that made Pannett's case for Acnotabs totally unacceptable.

In many ways the example of Acnotabs reflects the problems
that encouraged the FDA to push for the new legislation. In the
1950s and early 1960s agency personnel were becoming increasingly dissatisfied with their inability to distinguish publicly between effective and ineffective drugs. They feared that people
were endangering their health by taking worthless drugs, when
efficacious drugs were available. Sometimes the FDA attempted to
extend the safety provision to efficacy by claiming that "efficacy is
certainly a matter of safety when dependence is placed on the
drug for the treatment of a serious condition."[27] Moreover, the
agency found that the evidence in support of therapeutic efficacy
was often unsubstantiated, consisting primarily of "testimonials
from practicing physicians who casually tested experimental
drugs on their patients and were paid for their efforts." Supporting increased government control of the marketing of new drugs,
these spokespersons were particularly concerned that the FDA
could be forced to approve ineffective drugs because it lacked the
specific authority to reject them.[28] Such, certainly, was the case the
agency fought with Pannett over Acnotabs.

As early as 1958, the FDA publicly discussed the need for legislation requiring manufacturers to prove their claims for efficacy.[29]
When revisions to the law were proposed in 1961, testimony in
Congress supported the efficacy requirements. Physicians and
other interested parties insisted that "a collection of impressions,"
that is, clinical evidence gathered in the course of private practice, was insufficient evidence. In addition, it was claimed that
"modern therapeutics is too difficult and too dangerous for today's doctor to go it alone. He needs help."[30] The FDA was joined
by many others in its insistence on broad-based clinical trials. In

the same period, projects of the National Institutes of Health demonstrated its increasing support for clinical trials, which reflected the commitment of the research community to expanding trials.[31] And major pharmaceutical houses, such as Eli Lilly and Company, proudly announced that "the 'testimonial' type of clinical report is no longer acceptable. Information based on adequately controlled studies is demanded before the claims made by the pharmaceutical manufacturer are accepted."[32] By this time, Acnotabs exemplified an older standard of scientific evidence.

For many months the bill to revise the 1938 Food, Drug and Cosmetic Act languished in both houses of Congress, despite numerous rewritings. Then, in mid-1962, the thalidomide story broke in the *Washington Post.* In September 1960, the William S. Merrill Pharmaceutical Company had applied to the FDA for approval of thalidomide as a new product. Despite no clear evidence of danger, Dr. Frances Kelsey, the FDA examiner, kept returning the application to the manufacturer, requesting additional information before she would issue approval. By late 1961, in Europe thalidomide was identified as the cause of an alarming increase in the number of children born with a condition called phocomelia. (The term is derived from two Greek words meaning "seal" and "limb." In cases of phocomelia the arms of a fetus fail to grow completely, resulting in arms so short that the hands appear to extend from the shoulders; legs suffer a similar lack of development.) Meanwhile, the condition also appeared in this country in families who had purchased thalidomide in Europe or who had received the product as part of a U.S. trial that had released over 2.5 million tablets to more than 1,200 doctors. The news of the stricken children generated such support for new drug legislation that the enfeebled bill was reworked, and with the efficacy requirement included it quickly passed into law.[33]

The Kefauver-Harris Amendment to the bill required drug companies preparing a new product to submit to the FDA a plan for clinical trials, documentation of past animal and clinical trials, and the names and qualifications of the investigators. Uncontrolled studies conducted through the practices of private physicians would not suffice. Expert testimony was needed. The legislation itself defined what evidence was needed and delegated evaluation and decision making to scientific experts: "The term 'substantial evidence' means evidence consisting of adequate and well-controlled investigations, including clinical investigations, by experts qualified by scientific training and experience to evaluate the effectiveness of the drug involved, on the basis of which it could fairly and responsibly be concluded by such experts that the drug will have the effect it purports or is represented to have under the conditions of use prescribed, recommended, or suggested in the labeling or proposed labeling thereof."[34]

Clearly, Pannett did not have the data to satisfy the more rigorous standards of testing and efficacy demanded by Kefauver-Harris; it could not prove that its product cured acne. The company was forced to halt the sale of Acnotabs. The elevation of scientific expertise in legislation undercut the role of the layperson in evaluating scientific disputes over specific therapeutic claims. Questions of science do not remain within the narrow confines of a scientific community; they often lay at the center of issues of public policy.[35] The locus of authority for science shifts in American society. By the mid-1960s, the definition of science, of what constituted acceptable scientific practice, was established in the Kefauver-Harris Amendment. It removed certain decision making from the laity, placing it in the hands of scientific experts and rendering the judge's decision in the Acnotabs case moot.

Within the scientific community, choice between competing theories demands clear, unambiguous, generally accepted experimental results. If the results are open to different interpretations and if those different interpretations are dependent on different underlying principles, then interpretations at variance with orthodox science will be labeled at best incompetent and at worst quackery.[36] As we have seen, this is what happened to Linus Pauling. Though the FDA never went so far as to claim that Acnotabs was quackery, the agency did criticize Kelter's test from the standpoint of orthodox scientific theories and methodology. Kelter's recourse to alternative hypotheses, especially in light of his uncertain results, severely weakened his case in the eyes of orthodox scientists. The judge, however, had stood outside the scientific community. While accepting orthodoxy he at the same time was unwilling to deny the possibilities of Kelter's experiences. Government representatives, secure in their views, had no such problem. With the passage of the Kefauver-Harris Amendment, orthodox definitions of science gained political clout.

Contemporary science was the decisive factor in both the prosperity of Miles and the demise of Pannett. The promotion of One-A-Day pushed the results of popular science to a logical conclusion; vitamin pills could be useful even if a person appeared well-nourished. Those of Acnotabs reached beyond the limits of orthodox science; the evidence did not prove that the product cured acne. Miles's use of science worked because its claims were backed by references to current scientific publications, references the FDA and other detractors could question but not ignore. Pannett's scientific claims were hyperbole and they harkened back to an earlier empirical norm in science, a norm no longer credible. Though science held an esteemed position in popular culture, scientific rhetoric could not insure success.

# CHAPTER 6

# "Millions of Consumers Are Being Misled"

## The Food and Drug Administration and Consumer Protection

The Kefauver-Harris Amendment did not become the final arbiter of vitamin claims nor even settle the matter of vitamins for the Food and Drug Administration. The FDA positioned itself as the arbiter of conflicting scientific claims, a position that has not gone unchallenged. The agency's self-image was as a disinterested, unbiased spokesperson for science; many of its opponents, though, painted the FDA as a misguided interpreter of scientific results and even as a dupe of the medical and scientific establishment. Consumers who differed dramatically with the agency's views did not reject science. They continued to embrace its cultural authority and their interpretations of its findings. The FDA, however, acted as if it had a monopoly on science. As consumers, manufacturers, and members of the scientific community increasingly and publicly debated scientific results, the agency could not maintain its credibility.

True, using the scientific standards embedded in the legislation, the FDA could and did remove products such as Acnotabs from the market. The legislative definition of science gave the agency a more secure ground from which to police the growing vitamin industry. In the more than three decades since the Pannett case, the FDA has continued to monitor and prosecute vitamin products promoted with questionable claims. This case-by-case procedure could be quite time-consuming and costly, and

• • • • • • • • • • • • • • • • • • • • • • • • • • • • • • • • • • • • •

consequently the agency sought other mechanisms for control-ling the industry. The FDA's long struggle to establish categorical regulations brings into high relief the many scientific, political, and cultural factors that have given vitamins such honor and no-toriety in our consumer culture.

Vitamin supplementation has been argued in a variety of fo-rums. Popular magazines, newspapers, the trade press, medical journals, storefronts, courtrooms, the offices of government agen-cies, and advertisements in print, on radio, and on television all provided space for advocates of vitamins and their adversaries. These diverse arenas presented fragmentary views shaped by the medium, the audience, and competitors. In this cacophony of opinions and claims, the debate over the FDA regulation of vita-min supplements functioned as the focal point for scientific, med-ical, nutritional, economic, and political anxieties. The controversy illuminated the unequal power relations among the various fac-tions and underscored the different ways science was interpreted in American society.

The FDA asserted its vision of governmental regulation over vitamins in the 1940s, in the 1960s, and again in the 1970s. Each attempt met with greater and greater opposition. Fearing for their very existence, some vitamin producers and retail outlets mobilized concerned citizens to petition Congress, the president, and the FDA directly. The exalted position of the medical profes-sion was openly questioned: did physicians have the knowledge and expertise they claimed, and could they be trusted to advise on vitamin supplements? Modern methods of agriculture and food processing came under scrutiny: was the American diet healthful? Over it all lay the question of the role of government in U.S. soci-ety: what were the limits of a governmental agency's powers in protecting the consumer? When to protect and when to inform? Just how far could or should the FDA's mandate lead it to restrict products? How to weigh the relative risks and benefits of un-checked availability of vitamin supplements? Who should judge risks and benefits: industry, scientists, the government, or the con-sumer? The argument over the limits of FDA authority, leading to the Proxmire Amendment of 1976, demonstrates how lack of scientific consensus could affect a political solution. The fact that Congress once again debated the issue in the 1990s documents the intractability of the question. With each new scientific announcement relating to food, health, and micronutrients, the problem of the place of vitamins in American culture surfaces again and again.

Though resistance to the FDA's attempts to control vitamin products became very public in the 1960s and especially the 1970s, the agency had monitored the industry from the beginning.[1] In the 1930s it discouraged advertising claims that suggested vitamin products were necessary for good health; in the 1940s it discouraged food fortification; and in the 1950s it litigated vitamin and mineral products with particularly blatant health claims. The Acnotabs case notwithstanding, the agency was relatively unsuccessful in all these efforts.

Insisting that the average American diet contained sufficient micronutrients, the FDA took a major step toward the regulation of vitamins in 1940 when it proposed a set of labeling requirements for all vitamin and mineral products.[2] The new labels were a form of consumer education, providing information about the content of the product and the scientific basis for health claims for it. They had to include the rationale for any dietary claims made. They also had to state whether the vitamin level of the product matched the daily minimum requirement established by the FDA. Moreover, if the product contained ingredients that were not yet established as necessary for human nutrition, the label must clearly state this. On the whole, major pharmaceutical houses did not object strongly to the new labels, despite the cost of redesigning labels and formulae. They saw these regulations as eliminating less scrupulous competitors from the market. Soon, though, another branch of the government, the U.S. Army, undercut the FDA's stand against vitamin supplements. In 1941 soldiers serving in the northern outposts of Iceland and Alaska were issued vitamin tablets. The army declared that the tablets were necessary to maintain the troops' nutritional status. (Interestingly, articles in the contemporary media declared that commercial products making similar health claims would have been investigated by the FDA for mislabeling.)[3] Before the FDA could respond to objections and comments from industry and other interested parties, the effective date of the regulations was postponed indefinitely during a reorganization of regulatory agencies in the executive branch. The FDA did not propose specific vitamin regulations again until the 1960s.

When the FDA returned to the question of vitamin regulations, many of the concerns that had spurred its 1940s' efforts were still very evident. The popular press provided a useful forum for the agency to promote its views. For example, a 1959 article in *Good Housekeeping*, "Are We Taking Too Many Vitamins?" written by Ruth and Edward Brecher, discussed the four "myths" used to persuade consumers to purchase vitamin supplements. They then refuted this mythology with extensive quotations from FDA officials. The first myth was that all diseases were due to improper diet. True, the FDA admitted, there were deficiency diseases, but they were rarely encountered in the United States, and when they did occur, they should be treated by a physician, not by self-medication with vitamin supplements. The second myth concerned the question of soil depletion. FDA spokespersons denied that U.S. food was grown in poor soil; chemically fertilized soils produce nutritionally adequate food. Furthermore, soil deficiency did not result in disease, except in the case of iodine and goiter for which the remedy was simple: the use of iodized salt. The third myth was that modern food was overprocessed, stripping away the nutritional value. According to FDA officials, contemporary food processing preserved micronutrients and even improved manufactured foods such as flour, bread, and margarine with the addition of vitamins and minerals. The incongruity inherent in this position, that food contained sufficient nutrients, but adding nutrients made food better, was not discussed. Fourth was the myth of subclinical deficiencies, that a lack of vitamins could cause a general run-down feeling without any definite symptoms or specific cause: "According to the subclinical deficiency myth, anyone who has 'that tired feeling' or an ache or pain in almost any part of the body is probably suffering from a deficiency and needs to supplement his diet with some concoction or other. There is no reason whatever for believing that such vague symptoms are commonly due to subclinical vitamin or mineral deficiencies. Such symptoms may have many other causes." The Brechers also quoted FDA officials who insisted that regardless of advertising claims, vitamin preparations would not cure physical ailments such as asthma, alcoholism, cancer, and colds. People who believed such statements, the agency feared, would rely on self-medication, rather than seek appropriate medical advice.

The impact of articles such as these is difficult to judge. *Good Housekeeping* was a very popular magazine with a wide circulation, especially among middle-class consumers. Moreover, the article was abridged and reprinted in *Science Digest* and a month later in *Reader's Digest.*[4] Together these pieces undoubtedly spread the FDA's philosophy on vitamins to a wide audience and alerted many to the agency's reasoned opposition to supplementation. Yet at the same time, these articles provided support for vitamin supplementation as well. The authors noted that the U.S. produced a "wide range of nutritious foodstuffs" that "enables *most* people *most* of the time to meet *all* their vitamin and mineral needs through their regular meals" (emphasis in the original). They then listed exceptional cases such as babies, pregnant women, nursing mothers, people recovering from illness, and people on restricted diets. And also, "the individual who, through ignorance, poor eating habits, or emotional or physical illness, does not eat an adequate diet." Although, the Brechers hastened to add that it was preferable in such instances to correct one's diet, still they admitted that vitamin supplements were an alternative. Vitamin products, in effect, were insurance for an insufficient diet. Articles like this were typical. On the one hand, writers praised the American food supply and the American diet, dismissing the need for vitamin products; on the other hand, they cautioned that not everyone is eating well and advised some people to take vitamins for nutritional insurance.

The FDA did not see the issue that way; to the agency vitamin supplementation was simply another form of health quackery, and a very lucrative one at that. In this the FDA had the support of the American Medical Association, the leading organization of

• • • • • • • • • • • • • • • • • • • • • • • • • • • • • • • • • • • •

physicians in the country. For years the two groups worked in tandem to identify and prosecute excessive health claims on vitamin products.[5] In October 1961, they jointly sponsored a National Congress on Medical Quackery in Washington, D.C. Newspapers were quick to pick up on some of the most outrageous claims cited at the conference, especially claims dealing with vitamin products. George Larrick, FDA commissioner, was widely quoted for his contention that "millions of consumers are being misled" about their need for vitamin supplementation. He estimated that vitamin and health quackery cost half a billion dollars annually.[6]

The agency's goal was to protect the consumer both financially (unnecessary vitamins were a waste of money) and nutritionally (excessive intake of vitamins could be hazardous to one's health). As the example of Acnotabs demonstrates, agency procedures, which required case-by-case litigation, made prosecution of such products difficult and time-consuming. Thus, the regulations announced in June 1962 aimed to give the FDA a more effective and efficient means of controlling vitamin products.[7] Larrick believed that consumers lacked the information they needed to make reasoned choices; consequently, they were misled into thinking that their diets were "inadequate." This ignorance induced consumers to buy products loaded with "many times the daily requirement of most, if not all, of the nutrients" in the belief that each ingredient made "a significant addition to his customary diet." Larrick's description portrayed the consumer as a pawn, easily persuaded by advertising claims. New labeling standards would assure that consumers would have "complete information" about their purchases.[8] The regulations would allow labels to make claims only for nutrients "generally recognized as essential in human nutrition" and in amounts "likely to be of value." Of course, the FDA would make those judgments based on contemporary science.

As expected, manufacturers responded—vehemently. Not only industry but individual vitamin users filed objections. According to one report, the agency received 54,000 responses, of which 40,000 were postcards initiated by the National Health Federation, a group associated with nutritional supplement companies. The federation was not highly regarded by the FDA; several of

NHF's officers were from the more radical wing of the industry and had been convicted of making false claims for their products.[9] But elements of the mainstream pharmaceutical industry expressed concern as well. For example, Abbott Laboratories, which at the time sold thirty-three supplement products, complained that under the regulations, "virtually none" of its line could be marketed.

Given strong industry and consumer reaction and faced with enforcing an unpopular rule with a limited staff, the FDA shelved the regulations, though the agency continued its media campaign against the widespread use of vitamin supplements.[10] In its role as protector of the health of Americans, the FDA tried to convince consumers to reject vitamin supplements. Their admonishments apparently fell on deaf ears because over the years the industry continued to grow.[11]

In the face of its failure to change the buying habits of the public through education, the agency in June 1966 once again decided to regulate the market—this time by requiring that all vitamin and mineral supplements carry the infamous crepe label that would so enrage Miles and other pharmaceutical manufacturers.[12] Despite the evident controversy within the scientific community, the FDA had decided that scientific evidence for vitamin supplementation did not exist and that this should be indicated directly on the vitamin products sold to consumers.

The new rules also dealt with the content of vitamin products. The FDA found that the term "minimum daily requirement" (MDR) misled many consumers who assumed that if a little was good, more was better—a conclusion the agency flatly rejected. Instead of the MDR, the FDA proposed "recommended dietary allowance" (RDA) as the standard. The content level of vitamin products must henceforth be in line with established RDAs. In addition, the agency mandated the contents of multivitamin supplements: they were required to contain vitamins A, D, C, $B_1$, $B_2$, and niacin; they could include vitamins E, $B_6$, folic acid, pantothenic acid, and $B_{12}$. The rules also specified the maximum and minimum amounts of each vitamin. These standards would, the agency believed, protect the consumer in two ways. First, they established rational formulae for vitamin products; no longer would the consumer face a confusing array of merchandise with widely varying contents. Second, the requirements prevented the practice of loading supplements with less costly ingredients while providing little of the most expensive ones. It is critical to note that the rules affected most companies selling vitamin supplements at the time because almost all the products on the market would need to be altered.[13]

According to James Lee Goddard, then the FDA commissioner, the new rules were based on the best science of the day: "We read the scientific literature and we go to the best scientists in the United States. This is based on careful scientific evaluation." Though Goddard was convinced of the scientific basis for the regulations, he knew that there would be significant resistance. Manufacturers were the obvious dissenters, but scientists too were uncomfortable with the new rules.[14] Therefore, rather than allowing the standard thirty days for comments to be filed on proposed regulations, Goddard extended the comment period to sixty days. The agency was required to hold public hearings if so requested, and, not surprisingly, they were demanded.

The opposition to the FDA proposals quickly marshaled its strength. Whereas earlier proposals had had the support or at least the acquiescence of most major drug houses, the 1966 rules raised the ire of most pharmaceutical companies and organizations, as well as consumer groups. Miles Laboratories immediately objected. The crepe label in particular upset the company. Though agreeing that vitamins are present in foods, the company reiterated its nutritional insurance argument, insisting that "it is a myth that because nutritional foods are available, everyone routinely eats them in well-balanced meals." People have different personal preferences, and "many other factors beyond our control—including age, sex, psychological, medical, economic, geographic and vocational factors—affect when and how much we eat." The company's declarations that "as a practical matter for the general public, the only firm assurance of an adequate vitamin intake is to supplement one's food with a good-quality multiple vitamin," echoed its advertising theme.[15] And Miles was not the only major drug company to reject the FDA's proposals. By September, twelve pharmaceutical concerns, including Miles and the Pharmaceutical Manufacturers Association, Abbott Laboratories, Merck & Co., Pfizer & Co., Upjohn Company, and Wyeth Laboratories, had filed suit in federal court to prevent the FDA from implementing the new rules.[16]

Under heavy pressure, the FDA delayed the effective date of the regulations and scheduled public hearings for early 1967. Even before the hearings opened, the agency announced modifications to the proposed rules. Trying to meet objections to the "crepe label," the FDA presented a new label, which had now been softened to read: "Vitamin and minerals are supplied in abundant amounts by commonly available foods. Except for persons with special medical needs, there is no scientific basis for recommending routine use of dietary supplements."[17] But the agency would go no farther; it sustained other rules opposed by many consumers and manufacturers. Even modified, the regulations still mandated that multivitamin supplements had to contain certain ingredients and contain them at a level no greater and no less than that determined by the FDA. The agency continued to justify this decision on scientific grounds, explaining that "the permissible nutrient levels have been adapted by FDA from information in a report of the Food and Nutrition Board of the National Academy of Sciences-National Research Council, considered the foremost authority on nutrition in the United States."[18] The agency clearly intended, and stated, that most supplements then sold in the United States would need to be changed to conform to the published standards.

It took more than a year for the hearings to begin, in May 1968.[19] Goddard consistently complained about the "great misunderstanding" over the regulations and the hearings. He maintained that the agency was "not trying to keep people from buying vitamins. There is no intent to rule vitamins out of the market." He insisted that the rules were necessary for the protection of the consumer. Though he personally believed that vitamins were unnecessary, he doubted that vitamin supplements could ever be eliminated in a society so enamored with "pill-taking."[20] Others disagreed, most particularly vitamin manufacturers who feared that the crepe label was their death knell.

Kirkpatrick W. Dilling, general counsel of the National Association of Food Supplement Manufacturers, fiercely protested the FDA proposal, finding it to be based on false premises. He contended that there was no such thing as an ordinary or average diet; and that if there were, it would not automatically insure that "everyone receives excellent nutrition." Dilling complained not only about the rules, but also about the delay in hearings. During the postponement, he believed, the "agency has conducted a vicious nationwide campaign of 'trial by publicity,' intended to discredit the vitamin and food supplement industry."[21] Not certain that the industry would win the hearts and the minds of the American consumer through the popular media alone, he wanted hearings as soon as possible to give the industry a platform from which to combat the agency's attacks.

There were others, however, who would have preferred to delay the hearings still further. Some researchers were less certain than Goddard of the scientific basis for the regulations and they believed that more study was needed before the necessary evidence would be available for discussion. In July 1968, Frederick J. Stare, chair of the Department of Nutrition at the Harvard University School of Public Health, asked then–FDA Commissioner Herbert Ley to further postpone the hearings. "No one has really done their homework on this subject," according to Stare, who went on to enumerate activities he believed warranted a wait.

> The Recommended Dietary Allowances have been revised. The Council on Foods and Nutrition of the American Medical Association and the Food and Nutrition Board [of the National Academy of Science-National Research Council] are planning to "liberalize" their policy on enrichment and fortification. HEW [the U.S. Department of Health, Education, and Welfare] via Dr. Arnold Schaefer's office is starting to gather some "facts" via nutrition surveys in representative areas of the country on the extent and degree of malnutrition.[22]

These developments suggested that important new information would be forthcoming shortly. Stare did not want regulations based on incomplete results.

Other prominent nutritional scientists and physicians seconded Stare's request even after the hearings began.[23] Their letters to the FDA closely followed a call by the Mead Johnson Company for a recess "pending the availability of enough pertinent information to justify revision of the regulations." The company had asked scientists for their support of its request to postpone the hearings. Evidently a number of researchers and physicians agreed and wrote the FDA about their concern "at the waste of money and time of both industry and the Food and Drug Administration which the present hearings require."[24] For Calvin Woodruff, professor of pediatrics at the University of Missouri, there was no urgency forcing hasty hearings: "No great public health crisis in this area besets harm to the public—and further delay in the interest of scientific accuracy would seem justified."[25] Clearly the scientific community was not uniformly backing the FDA's drive for vitamin regulation at this time, finding such control premature and unnecessary.

Ley responded to such requests with administrative rationale. He explained that the hearing procedure was mandated by the law. But it was not only procedural regulations that guided the hearings. Ley also maintained that in the evolving field of nutrition there would always be new studies. If the FDA waited for these studies to be completed, it would never convene the hearings.[26] He accepted as a fact of life that current research would provide new information probably "dictat[ing] a change in the regulations established, [such that] these changes can be and will undoubtedly have to be made."[27]

In seeking to establish scientifically based regulation to govern vitamins, the FDA had to contend with the objections of the industry and the uncertainty of the scientific community. It also faced public opposition from another governmental agency that provided data directly contradicting the FDA's claims. Just as the hearings were finally opening in 1968, a U.S. Department of Agri-

• • • • • • • • • • • • • • • • • • • • • • • • • • • • • • • • • • • • • • • •

culture study reported that half of the households in its national survey had diets that failed to meet the recommended dietary allowances of one or more micronutrients.[28] Quickly vitamin companies used the USDA survey to argue for the need for vitamin supplementation among the American populace. The research also received wide play in the general news media and in specialty journals such as *Organic Gardening and Farming*. Shortly after the survey was released, editor J. I. Rodale gleefully cited its results to demonstrate the need for vitamin supplementation. As reported by him and numerous other journal articles, the study showed that the American diet had declined seriously over the last decade. In 1955, a similar survey concluded that 60 percent of Americans had "good" diets, 15 percent had "poor" ones. In 1965, the percentage of those with "good" diets dropped to fifty, while now 20 percent were in the "poor" category. Moreover, "undernutrition" was evident among the "so-called healthy population," as well as the aged and the chronically ill. This was not a question of gross vitamin deficiencies—surveys were not uncovering rickets or scurvy or beriberi in large numbers—but a question of possible subclinical deficiencies caused by inadequate vitamin intake. For Rodale, the reasons were clear: deficient soil produced nutritionally deficient foods and overprocessing stripped modern convenience foods of their nutritional values.[29] Even the American Medical Association, a staunch supporter of the FDA, and the National Academy of Sciences admitted that food processing had its nutritional problems. In a joint statement, the AMA and the NAS recommended research into food production, processing, and storage in order to devise methods for retaining food's nutritional value. They even suggested fortifying foods whose nutritive content was lost through refining and other processing.[30] Whether they agreed or disagreed with Rodale's analysis and the AMA-NAS report, many commentators over the next few years repeated the USDA statistics in their fight against the FDA's stand on vitamin supplementation and the argument about overprocessing.

Other opponents found evidence of nutritional insufficiency in different studies. While Goddard had claimed that $500 million was wasted annually on vitamins and other so-called health foods,

Stanley N. Gershoff, of the Nutrition Department of the Harvard School of Public Health, declared such statements "absolutely absurd." Gershoff's survey of nutritional studies conducted between 1950 and 1968 disclosed that the American diet was deteriorating and many people were taking in less than half the recommended daily allowances of many vitamins. Biochemical indices showed that deficiencies were common. His conclusion clashed dramatically with that of the FDA: "In short, the people studied, primarily middle-class, could effectively utilize vitamin supplements."[31] Scientists such as Gershoff envisioned the use of routine vitamin supplementation, even among those with supposedly better diets.

Given such differences of opinion even within the professional groups from which the FDA supposedly drew its support, it was expected that the hearing process would be lengthy. The hearings began on 21 May 1968 before hearing examiner David H. Harris. Following standard regulatory procedures, Harris was to gather all the evidence and to submit a report to the commissioner of the FDA, who would make a tentative decision. Exceptions to this decision could be filed before the commissioner announced the final decision, which was then subject to court appeal. In his 1970 exposé of the agency, *The Chemical Feast*, James S. Turner determined that up to that point the FDA had spent nearly $200,000, compiled 26,000 pages of testimony, and committed thousands of FDA staff-hours to the operation. To what result? he asked. The FDA's attempts to refute claims of malnutrition and undernutrition in the United States had become "increasingly embarrassing." He noted that "scientists and researchers in the field of nutrition have been appalled by the FDA's activities in the vitamin field almost since they began."[32] Turner pointed out that one of the most unusual aspects of the vitamin hearings and the push for the crepe label was that the FDA managed to alienate both consumers and industry. The agency also alienated many scientists whose support it needed.

In reviews of Turner's book, others expressed concerns about basic problems within the FDA and about its handling of vitamin supplementation. They believed these were indicative of the Agency's difficult relationship with scientists. *Science* undertook a

• • • • • • • • • • • • • • • • • • • • • • • • • • • • • • • • • • • • • • • • •

careful analysis of the book, explaining that *The Chemical Feast* was produced by a student task force working under consumer advocate Ralph Nader. Conceding that the investigators presumably expected to find "how the system had gone wrong," the reviewer was not surprised that the book "reads more like an indictment than like a balanced appraisal." Yet the evidence provided was convincing: "The FDA is unquestionably in need of a major overhaul." *Science* cited the push for the regulation of vitamins as an example of "almost incredible . . . bungling." The review noted, as had the book, that the FDA claimed support from the National Academy of Science–National Research Council for the crepe label. But the agency had altered the levels of the recommended daily allowances established by the NAS-NRC committee headed by William Sebrell, and so Sebrell joined in the censure of the FDA-proposed rules.[33]

In the early 1970s, the FDA found itself under attack from other quarters as well. These criticisms questioned the scientific credibility of the FDA's decisions. Take, for example, the controversy over vitamin C. The FDA had included vitamin C—ascorbic acid—on its 1959 GRAS ("generally recognized as safe") list of food chemicals. As the GRAS title suggests, food additives on the list are legally exempt from the safety testing demanded of other chemicals before they are allowed in the food supply. When Linus Pauling and his adherents in the late 1960s were calling for massive doses of vitamin C to prevent colds, FDA officials began to question vitamin C's GRAS rating.[34] Because of all the discussion, the agency even considered removing ascorbic acid from the GRAS list entirely; its reconsideration of the issue made it appear that science, at least the FDA's science, was not omniscient. This dispute received much attention in the popular press. Those who believed that the FDA's stand on vitamin supplementation was wrong could point to the vitamin C turnabout as another example of the insufficiency or changeability of scientific evidence.

By 1971, the FDA was no closer to vitamin regulation than it had been in 1966. Vitamin supplements with extravagant claims still abounded. In order to make its policy more efficient and effective, the FDA had proposed rigorous categorical regulations.

The "crepe label" made plain the agency's position: the American diet was sufficient and vitamin supplements were not necessary. The label would thus inform consumers who might have been misled by promotional campaigns. The FDA saw the label as consumer education; but, for pharmaceutical manufacturers and some scientists, the label was the most ominous and problematic aspect of the proposal. Hearings on the proposed regulations extended for nearly two years, with more than a hundred experts and vitamin advocates who spoke against all or part of the proposals and thirty-two government witnesses who spoke in its support; their testimony pitted one interpretation of the scientific data against another. In the words of one analyst, the 32,000 pages of testimony read like a debate between "government medical sleuths and nutrition experts against health-food enthusiasts, the food and drug industries and other nutrition experts."[35] At the very least, the FDA misjudged the level of scientific consensus on the question of vitamin supplementation; at the worst, the agency ignored the disagreement among nutritionists and physicians. At any rate, public media highlighted the scientific dissension. Was the American diet nutritionally sufficient or were Americans malnourished? Did the American diet contain all the required nutrients? These questions were raised over and over throughout the hearings.[36] The debate over the American diet alerted the public to differing claims within the scientific arena and lowered confidence in the FDA.

Other arguments surfaced as well. Members of the health-food industry, both manufacturers and independent store owners, claimed that the FDA was intent on putting them out of business. In fact Goddard had earlier boasted that most vitamin products on the market would disappear under the regulations.[37] Also, limiting the potencies of vitamin products to the recommended daily allowance was worrisome to advocates of megadosing. If, as the FDA proposed, vitamin C sold only in 100-milligram tablets, people would have to ingest as many as 100 tablets, which would tend to discourage users. The extensive objections showed that the FDA's goals were still far from accomplished.

By 1973, having digested the many, many pages of objections

and comments, the FDA issued another set of proposed regulations for vitamin supplements. FDA commissioner Alexander
Schmidt then announced that "the new regulations are based on
the best and broadest scientific evidence."[38] Once again, the FDA
justified its vitamin rules on scientific consensus. And still the proclaimed consensus did not exist. Many of the same complaints
heard in the 1940s and 1960s were repeated in opposition to the
proposals in the 1970s. There was still concern over widespread
malnutrition and subclinical vitamin deficiencies, even among
the supposedly well-nourished middle-class consumer. The
charges that physicians were insensitive to consumers' vitamin
needs and lacked the knowledge to understand deficiencies were
repeated. In addition, the argument for "freedom of choice"
gained in prominence. This theme had surfaced in earlier debates, but had not dominated the controversy. In the mid-1970s,
individual consumers, congressional representatives, industry
spokespersons, and even scientists returned over and over to the
singular importance of choice. In cases such as vitamin supplementation, they argued, in which experts differed dramatically,
the government did not have the right to dictate which products
the public could or should purchase. In an age that saw an out-
pouring of publications promoting self-help movements and support groups of all kinds, the argument of choice held great power.

In the 1973 rules, gone were the crepe label and the recipes for
standard vitamin products. In their place, the FDA divided vitamin products into three categories. Those containing less than 50
percent of the RDA were named foods; those between 50 and 150
percent of the allowance were dietary supplements; and products
of greater than 150 percent RDA were considered drugs. For the
FDA, the term dietary supplement meant products used by consumers as insurance against irregular or poor eating habits, not
for the treatment of disease. The intent of the new classification
scheme was, in Schmidt's words, to "insure more and better information to guide the consumer in making [nutritional] decisions."[39]
The agency returned to its earlier role of consumer educator, providing the information consumers needed to make choices within
limits defined by the FDA.

Unlike the 1960s regulations, the 1973 rules did not limit manufacturers to specific combinations of vitamins nor specific levels of potency. Products that went well beyond the RDA, however, were open to further FDA scrutiny as drugs. It was this last element of the regulations that attracted the most resistance. Advocates of megadosing obviously were concerned that consumers would not be able to purchase the desired dosages. For example, under the new rules, vitamin C tablets could be sold as dietary supplements in potency of up to ninety milligrams. (At this time the RDA for vitamin C was sixty milligrams.) Higher potencies would be labeled as drugs. In the early months of discussion, the FDA had not clarified whether or not consumers would need prescriptions to purchase higher doses. Many consumers rejected the need to see a physician before buying their vitamins. Cost alone would become a major hurdle. Moreover, megadosing consumers believed that they knew more about nutrition than physicians who usually rejected the use of massive doses of vitamins. There was an awkward alternative to physician's prescription: if manufacturers continued to produce vitamin C in potencies of ninety milligrams or less, then the consumer could ingest more tablets. Though consumers and health enthusiasts complained about this scenario as well, the FDA defended its regulations with the claim that "there is the possibility that there may be some inconvenience to the consumer, but we are not limiting his access to those vitamins."[40] But it was the "inconvenience" and the FDA power it represented that distressed megadose proponents.

Even when categorized as a drug, a product was not necessarily sold only by prescription; however, the controls on drugs were significantly more stringent than those governing food supplements. Under the 1960s amendments to the Food, Drug and Cosmetics Act, manufacturers were required to demonstrate the safety and the efficacy of drugs. These standards would make it much more difficult for vitamin products to pass FDA muster.

By the 1970s, new major adversaries of the FDA emerged. The National Health Federation (NHF) feared that the new rules would "wipe out an industry" and anticipated a lengthy court battle if the agency put the rules into effect. The organization had

• • • • • • • • • • • • • • • • • • • • • • • • • • • • • • • • • •

been involved in the earlier debates, but its leaders did not gain prominence until the 1970s. Clinton Miller, Washington lobbyist for NHF, likened the FDA's proposal to Prohibition: "These regulations have been compared to the Volstead Act, and when you take away a man's beer and his vitamins, you're in for some real trouble."[41] Moreover, of increasing significance in the 1970s controversy was the individual consumer: people who felt threatened by the proposals and feared loss of their vitamin supplements voiced their concerns in the offices of the agency and Congress.

These issues were not problems for everyone, and the FDA was not without its supporters. Many manufacturers accepted the new proposed rules. Bulk producers of vitamins felt that their business would not be affected. Even before the official announcement of the proposals, manufacturers of daily vitamin tablets, such as Miles Laboratories, declared that the rules would have little affect on their products. They concluded that the regulations were "aimed at irresponsible vitamin producers who are promising the sky with high doses."[42] Though the earlier rules had directly threatened the product lines of all manufacturers, these new rules necessitated only minor changes in their merchandise. The proposed rules not only allow their products, they also curtailed some of their more aggressive competitors.

Some consumer groups, such as the American Association of Retired Persons–National Retired Teachers Association, applauded the agency's actions. They held that the regulations were intended to "to protect consumers from being misled" into buying "unnecessary and useless products."[43] They agreed wholeheartedly with Schmidt that "the single and most important purpose and effect of the regulations is to require full and honest labeling and fair promotion of vitamin and mineral products as the basis for a more informed consumer choice."[44] "Informed" and "choice" were words repeated often in the debate. Everyone agreed that consumers needed information and should be free to make their own choices. Questions arose over who determined what was sufficient information and what limits were needed for safety.

The Health Research Group (HRG), associated with Ralph

Nader, put its weight behind the FDA's proposed rules as well. Admitting that they "often disagree with the way FDA handles dietary matters," spokespersons for the HRG nevertheless found themselves "sympathetic to its restrictions on vitamin sales." Nutritional problems probably did exist in the United States, but vitamin supplementation was not the answer, according to the HRG. For one thing, there were many vitamin products with unproven health claims. In addition, the safety testing of large doses remained undone.[45] The lack of scientific data required that the government control vitamin products, potential malnutrition notwithstanding. To the FDA and the HRG the scientific knowledge available was insufficient for unbridled informed consumer choice, and therefore the FDA needed to provide some restrictions, for the health and safety of the American public.

The disagreement among consumer advocates reflected the lack of unanimity among scientists. While the AARP-NRTA and the HRG aligned themselves with the FDA, other Naderites condemned the agency for its stand. On the one hand, agency supporters believed that, since the data were insufficient to judge healthfulness, these products should be restricted for the sake of consumer protection. On the other hand, *Chemical Feast* author James S. Turner maintained that because of the lack of clear scientific evidence, the FDA was in no position to mandate rules for the sale of vitamins. In his eyes, "the difficulty stems from the fact that the FDA is attempting to set national nutritional policy by Government regulation before any consensus on what that policy should be has developed."[46]

Lack of scientific evidence did not undermine faith in a scientific solution to the vitamin controversy. Both supporters and opponents considered science to be the arbiter of the question. But in the case of vitamins, science did not provide clear, unambiguous results. Consequently both sides used the very lack of scientific consensus to defend their own stands and to accuse their opponents of scientific ignorance.[47] Consumers themselves used the uncertainty of orthodox science to defend their right to choose.

# CHAPTER 7

# "Preserve Our Health Freedom"
## Science in Consumer Politics

Consumers themselves were not silent or passive while agents of industry, science, and government loudly proclaimed what the American public needed. Consumers spoke decisively with their wallets, fueling the growth of the vitamin industry. They petitioned Congress and they berated the Food and Drug Administration. Consumers castigated FDA officials for their arrogant claims about the ignorance and duplicity of the American public. They did not reject science but insisted that government officials listen to the experiences of families and individuals, to their interpretations of science, and to their faith in vitamins. Despite the agency's assurances that it was following the best scientific thinking of the day and despite its promise that the proposed rules would merely give the public more and better information, consumers believed that the FDA was determined to take vitamin supplements off the market. Confident in its stand, the FDA was blind to the strength of its opposition, as well as to the power of scientific disagreement to shape the public's view of vitamin supplementation and the depth of consumers' commitment to their vitamins.

Consumers vented their anger in letters to the FDA, to their congressional representatives, and to the president. As early as 1973, Commissioner Alexander Schmidt estimated that "tens of thousands of letters on the subject had been written to the agency and Congress."[1] Consumers may have been rationalizing their faith in vitamins with selective use of scientific evidence, but their letters reflected and reinforced the debate among scientists, manufacturers, and government officials. They made the controversy over vitamins less theoretical and less abstract. Their concerns put a personal face on the issue of vitamins in American society. At the same time, Congress entered the fray directly with a series of House and Senate hearings that placed the FDA and its proposals under closer scrutiny. The letters and congressional debates echoed many of the arguments heard earlier about the American diet and the need for vitamin supplementation. But now, the debate centered on the argument for choice, namely the consumer's right to choose vitamin products without government interference. Both opponents and supporters of the FDA exalted the importance of consumer choice. On the one side, the proposed regulations would insure that consumers could make intelligent choices among rational products based on scientific results. In other words, control of products enhanced consumer choice; restriction equaled protection. On the other side, such protection was unnecessarily inhibiting and paternalistic; only unrestricted product availability could insure consumers' choice. In an era that saw people marching in the streets for civil rights, women's rights, and welfare rights, the argument of choice was potent.

Angry consumers wrote the FDA; worried consumers wrote the FDA; frustrated consumers wrote the FDA. They had heard, either through a newspaper article, or radio program, or magazine story, or at their local health food store that the FDA would limit their access to vitamin products. They wanted the agency to know that they did not like that. FDA officials frequently claimed that the health food and supplement industries stirred up opposition to the proposed regulations. They pointed to the form letters and petitions prepared by organizations such as the National Health Federation. The agency typically characterized consumers as mindlessly following the suggestions of unscrupulous health enthusiasts. FDA files did fill with form letters, some of which were preprinted and some of which were handwritten copies. Consumers who sent in their own letters also repeated some of the same phrases popular in form letters. Yet from the number and range of letters in the FDA archives, it is clear that correspondents were not just following industry leaders. The issue of vitamin supplementation touched many who felt compelled to express their anger and anxiety to the responsible officials. While some writers utilized the forms provided by interested organizations, many others wrote from personal conviction about their own experiences. Some writers sent neatly typed letters with the argumentation carefully spelled out in detail; some sent long, handwritten, rambling letters. Others sent in brief, one or two sentence letters and postcards. Most correspondents wrote as concerned citizens; some identified themselves as professionals, professors, biochemists, nutritionists, retirees, and parents. They were convinced that the FDA rules would limit the availability of vitamin pills or make them unnecessarily expensive. And vitamin pills, they knew from personal experience and from scientific experts, were necessary for their health and the health of their families. They were defending their belief in vitamins from unreasonable government encroachment.

The archives of the FDA contain many petitions sent in opposition to the agency's proposals. Typically these preprinted forms protested that the FDA was expanding its reach into the homes of American citizens. They bemoaned the "bureaucratic encroachments upon our individual rights to determine what foods should be included in our diets, and to purchase nutritionally recognized vitamins without MEDICAL PRESCRIPTION, as we have done for many years with satisfactory results." When sent to members of Congress, the petitions would remind the addressee that "we intend to register our protests at the polls next November unless action is taken to curb" the FDA's actions.[2] Members passed these short and to-the-point appeals on to the agency.

The magnitude of consumers' convictions is clearest in the many, many letters received by the agency directly. A characteristic example was from a resident of Palm Springs, California, in the late 1960s.[3] Her letter reflected the personal commitment of many vitamin users and their interpretation of consumers' rights.

"We are among the many thousands who have serious and major nutritional deficiencies and health problems," she informed the FDA. She then enumerated her concerns: "Of necessity we must depend on hi-potency vitamin and mineral food supplements to literally help sustain health and life. Furthermore, many of us cannot afford to go to a Doctor for a prescription each time we need a new supply of hi-potency vitamins. Commissioner Goddard's very limited potency vitamins would be inadequate to our cases, as well as that of many others." Were vitamins necessary for her health? The FDA would probably insist that her vitamin needs could be supplied through an adequate diet, but the writer was convinced that she needed dietary supplements. She considered Goddard's actions outrageous and beyond his authority: "What right has FDA Commissioner Goddard to dictate regarding the needs of millions of Americans whose needs and conditions he does not even know? Surely no legitimate minded medical Doctor would prescribe for patients he has never seen or tested as he is trying to do."

The writer believed that vitamins were good and necessary for her and for others, though she clearly was not worried about the classic vitamin deficiency diseases like rickets and beriberi. She also knew that cigarettes and alcohol were harmful. In an earnest query repeated by many other correspondents, she asked: "Why not better limit the use and consumption of cancer causing, death dealing cigarettes (all tobacco) and alcoholic beverages, a really worth while need and cause?" Instead of wasting time and money to control vitamins, which to her mind were healthful, the FDA should use its authority to attack items recognized as unhealthy. Though the FDA and its supporters might dismiss her poignant plea to "preserve our Health Freedom" as a reflection of the National Health Federation's philosophy, the writer clearly believed that the agency's actions were putting her health and freedom in jeopardy. And her demands were repeated time and time again in the letters received by the agency.

Correspondents were mindful of the controversies surrounding the scientific claims made by the FDA to support the proposed regulations. They dramatized these arguments with observations from their personal health histories. One C.P.A. from Buffalo chided the agency for using the Recommended Daily Allowances. He reminded the FDA that the Food and Nutrition Board had developed RDAs for healthy persons, which limited their usefulness. For example, for years he and his family had been taking a common "one-a-day multiple vitamin" which included 200 milligrams of vitamin C and other vitamins also in excess of the recommended levels. He argued that "*it is important to emphasize and re-emphasize that no scientists or member of the Food and Drug Administration contends that there is any detrimental affect whosoever from dosages in excess of the recommended daily allowances which they are seeking to impose as ceiling and maximum.*"[4] In other words, doses in excess of RDAs helped maintain one's health.

Such doses were also backed by scientists who wrote the FDA in protest over the proposed regulations. One researcher associated with the Department of Health, Education and Welfare's National Heart and Lung Institute was particularly impressed with the studies documenting the positive effects of vitamin C "on health when given in gram quantities." He did not believe that one or two grams should be considered excessive. Moreover, he argued that "the concept of RDA seems to ignore the wide variations in individual metabolism. However if an RDA for vitamin C is necessary, I think it should be 2,000 mg. day." This researcher, and many other correspondents, also disagreed with the FDA about the sufficiency of the average American diet. Rather, he believed that much ill-health was directly attributable to poor nutrition, naming atherosclerosis, a major cause of death, as a nutritional disease, and linking nutrition and cancer. Given this connection, he proposed the need to revise totally our notions of the average diet. "I say, let the so-called food faddists experiment; anything is probably better than the present diet high in calories, carbohydrates, and carcinogens."

In his response, Commissioner Schmidt attempted to disentangle the many factors noted by the researcher. On the specific issue of vitamin C, he felt that the research was incomplete. Until there was more evidence, he would continue to accept the board's RDA. Schmidt dismissed the connection between atherosclerosis and nutrition as "overly simplistic." He did agree that the typical American diet needed improvement. In a curious turn of phrase, he insisted that the FDA did not say that the average American diet leads to good health, rather that "a typical well-balanced American diet does not lead to deficiencies that need to be made up for by taking dietary supplements, vitamins, etc."[5] The commissioner's annoyance is clear in his response, but the arguments presented by this correspondent are typical of what the agency received.

The HEW scientist sought to convince the agency to recognize that new knowledge might well change our outlook on vitamins; other letter writers reminded the FDA about how rapidly nutritional science was changing. One Tacoma, Washington, resident used evolving science and personal experience to lambaste the FDA's position on vitamins. He explained that vitamin E was for many years listed as one for which "no need in human consumption [has been] established." Recently nutritionists had established a maximum of thirty International Units per day, while larger doses were classified as therapeutic. Yet, "for your information, my wife and I have been taking 200 to 300 units of E a day for years and are in excellent health and have been for years, according to our Doctor."[6] To this writer, the agency's scientific claims meant little in light of rapidly changing scientific standards and in comparison to his family's health.

Knowing that vitamin supplementation was frequently associated with food faddism, other writers (unlike the HEW research) explicitly distanced themselves from the more radical fringe elements. As one woman put it: "Though I've read books on nutrition I am no 'vitamin nut.'"[7] These vitamin users did not insist on the efficacy or even the need for megadoses, but they wanted to make sure that they could continue to purchase their chosen vitamins. Even moderate supplementers, evidently, felt threatened by the proposed FDA regulations. These letters typically came from parents who were convinced that their family's health depended on some vitamin supplementation. They did not see vitamins as always necessary, but rather as insurance for times when family members might not be eating well. "Yes, we have vitamin bottles

• • • • • • • • • • • • • • • • • • • • • • • • • • • • • • • • •

on our breakfast table," wrote one woman from Pittsburgh. "But just as some days my family does not eat their 'standard American diet,' so too on many days I forget to pass out the vitamins. I think it evens itself out in the long run." Given the way she used vitamin products, she requested that the FDA be concerned that "multi-vitamin & mineral mixtures are well balanced."[8]

Other letter writers were accepting of certain aspects of FDA work. Both praising vitamins and reprimanding the agency for trying to restrict their availability, some correspondents outlined what they saw as the FDA's crucial role in vitamin regulation. Archetypical was a letter from Rockport, Maine, which both chastised the agency for its proposals and instructed it on its appropriate sphere. Having taken vitamins for twenty years and maintained excellent health, the writer insisted that it was neither the agency's right nor duty to limit the availability of vitamin products. Which did not mean that the FDA should have no involvement in the industry; after all, the agency was charged with protecting the health of citizens: "Naturally the purity of preparations should come under control; also companies should be required to correctly state the amount of each nutrient on the label; but beyond that the government should have no jurisdiction." If the FDA was truly concerned about the health of Americans, it should focus its attention on cigarettes, stimulants, and depressants. The FDA had an important role to play in protecting the health of the country, but not in the control of vitamins. If vitamins were a waste of money, which the writer did not think they were, then it was up to the individual whether or not to waste money. "You don't try to regulate the sale of liquor because it is a waste of the individual's money!" noted the correspondent. "We have as much right to our vitamins as others do to their liquor."[9]

More often, letter writers had little or nothing good to say about the FDA's interference with their vitamin supplementation. Much of the correspondence repeated the charge that the American diet was deficient, frequently citing the studies discussed in the public media. The U.S. Department of Agriculture survey was mentioned over and over again. Yet many letters explained that Americans' nutrition need not be poor if the FDA "would start doing your job and if Government started to educate people on proper nutrition, but the Food Processors are a mighty big lobby in Washington, aren't they?" queried "a concerned American."[10] Instead of regulating vitamins, many correspondents commented, the FDA should look to other, more pressing health concerns.

Consumers demanded that the agency do more to control the healthfulness and safety of the food supply, which they believed was compromised with additives. As early as the 1930s, food enrichment had begun in this country, first with the addition of vitamin D and later other vitamins. For example, scientists claimed that 90 percent of the vitamin $B_1$ in bread is lost from the flour through the milling process. Mortality rates did not reflect this malnutrition, but, they concluded, untold numbers of people were walking around with subclinical vitamin deficiencies. In the 1940s, first the states and then the federal government passed enrichment laws mandating that manufacturers replace nutrients processed out of food.[11] Though the FDA was concerned about the haphazard fortification of so many products, by the outset of World War II the agency accepted the idea of enriching flour and bread as a way to compensate for potential nutritional problems. After the war, a growing chemical industry produced many new chemical additives designed to enhance the nutritional value and shelf life of modern food products.[12] In the early 1950s, the Delaney congressional hearings investigated the industry, detailing the extent to which foods were manipulated in processing and production and documenting the range of additives. Evidence presented there, and well-publicized in the popular press, highlighted differences of opinion among scientists about the safety of many additives. More significantly, the hearings also showed the FDA as a weak agency lacking the power to protect public health and safety. New legislation increased control of the food supply, but the hearings had further lowered consumer confidence in the FDA.[13]

Worried about the nutrition of their families, some vitamin users demanded that the FDA instead ban additives that "do nothing to improve food nutritionally" since "many like sodium nitrate can be harmful."[14] Another correspondent was "very angry" about the FDA's stand on vitamin supplementation. She pointed out that "we have numerous *harmful* chemicals which you allow to be added to our foods," so why was the agency focusing on vitamins?[15] "If H.E.W. is so concerned about our health," asked another letter writer, "why is it suitable to add preservatives, stabilizers, flavors, colors and sweeteners to our vitamins and minerals?"[16] Writers frequently instructed agency officials: "If you really want to do something worth while take the additives and perservities [*sic*] out of food."[17] These people did not deny the FDA's role in the protection of public health, nor the value of scientific evidence, but they most definitely disagreed with the agency's interpretation of hazards. The arguments they had heard about the composition of the American food supply led them to doubt the safety of processed food and to embrace their vitamins even more vigorously.

The debate over the GRAS list also entered into the correspondence files. One particularly irate writer accused the FDA of waffling on the list: "I also read that the FDA permits a total of 674 additives to food which are 'generally recognized as safe.' However, the FDA is now 'reviewing the safety of all these substances.' This means, of course, that the FDA really does not know whether or not the 'safe' classification is correct. . . . I believe that these additives are allowed for economic considerations, certainly do nothing to promote good health in the population, and may be the cause of the nation's many ills."[18] Some applauded the agency's willingness to revise the GRAS with current data; they saw it as openmindedness, the appropriate approach to an evolving science. To others it was further evidence of the uncertainty in the field. Thus it further weakened the FDA's position. If what the FDA had classified as "generally safe" was now questionable, why should people believe the FDA when it branded vitamins unsafe? Where was the data to support that designation? Many people took vitamins, took them in massive doses, and felt better for it, claimed letter writers. If the FDA was so sure that vitamins were injurious, the agency was obligated to demonstrate concrete evidence of harm. One concerned correspondent explained: "It has been said that you are going to take away my right to take vitamins. Well, you might as well have sentenced me to capital pun-ishment! I have been using vitamins for five years, and they have done nothing less than given me a rebirth that has made me feel, at times, like a mortal messiah!"[19]

Though the FDA denied it, many consumers believed that the proposed regulations would make vitamin products inaccessible except by prescription. In form letters and in personalized letters, the agency explained to concerned consumers that supplements in excess of 150 percent RDA were taken as drugs, not nutrients. "FDA does not want to ban such uses, but does believe that such high levels should be taken under proper medical supervision," the agency informed consumers.[20] But consumers persisted in be-lieving otherwise. Letter after letter to the agency deplored the FDA's proposals and pleaded with the agency not to take away vitamins, not to require that consumers see physicians to get pre-scriptions for products they used every day for their health.

Because of the volume of mail, the agency sometimes was forced to respond with form letters. Some consumers read these preprinted letters as confirmation of the FDA's arrogance and felt they deserved a more individualized answer to their highly per-sonalized correspondence. They would return the form letters with scathing comments about the FDA's lack of concern for their issues. To mitigate this ill feeling, the agency explained that it received a tremendous amount of correspondence, much of which was "preprinted and really did not provide us with much information about the correspondent's personal views." All letters were read, the FDA assured consumers, but economics precluded answering each one individually. As Gerald F. Mayer, director of the FDA Office of Legislative Services explained to one indignant correspondent, "It costs something less than $1 to respond to a general type of inquiry with preprinted information materials. It can cost up to $20 to respond to each letter received with an individual reply. I would hope that a concerned consumer like yourself would be equally concerned at reducing the cost to the Federal Government when a preprinted response can adequately explain an issue."[21] Sometimes even this rationale did not satisfy consumers. And as the number of letters continued to increase, the FDA resorted to sending preprinted postcards in response to consumers' inquiries. The brief, three-sentence message merely thanked the correspondents for writing and informed the recipients that their opinions would be passed on to the hearing clerk.

In addition to the influx of form letters prepared by representatives of the health food industry, correspondence to the FDA over their proposed regulation of vitamin products contained a wide range of opinions and experiences. Some presented the agency with scientific data about the benefits of vitamin supplementation, some argued about the sufficiency of the American diet, some explained vehemently how the health of their families depended upon the availability of vitamin products, some were incensed at the thought of needing a prescription to buy their daily vitamins, and many letters combined several of these issues. But one point dominated the letters from consumers. The overwhelming majority of correspondents indicted the FDA for its paternalistic attitude, calling the vitamin regulations an extreme example of "Big Brotherism." Over and over letter writers accused the agency of "treating the American people like children."[22] A few were willing to acknowledge the possibility that excessive vitamins might someday be proven to be harmful. "If the government feels certain vitamins in excess *may* be harmful," asked one writer, "why not merely require a warning label like cigarettes?"[23] Another correspondent identified himself as "a user of food supplements and as a citizen appalled by this chilling example of patronizing, daddy-knows-best arrogance."[24] Still others castigated the proposed rules as "arbitrary and arrogant."[25]

The FDA, of course, did not see itself as arrogant or paternalistic, and it did not understand this consumer perspective. Time after time, in newspapers and in hearing rooms and in letters to consumers, the agency explained that the proposed regulations were devised to "preserve every citizen's freedom to choose whatever safe foods he may wish to consume,"[26] and "to help consumers make wiser decisions involving their health."[27] This, then, was the crux of the controversy. The FDA believed that it could best protect the consumer by restricting product availability. There was no conclusive scientific data to convince the agency of the effectiveness of vitamin supplementation. Therefore, in its opinion, these products were at best useless and a waste of money, at worst harmful. Logically then, consumer protection mandated controlling the market of these worthless, dangerous products.

Consumers interpreted the situation differently. The very lack of definitive evidence, they concluded, made the FDA's action unwarranted. After all, their personal experiences told them that vitamins were effective and necessary. A resident of Detroit instructed the agency on the importance of vitamins. She and her husband had suffered from ill health until she read Adelle Davis, a popular nutrition writer, and began experimenting with high-potency products. "After years of reading and experimenting, I have FINALLY arrived at a supplementation that affords us the ultimate in well-being and my husband and I, although now in our mid-thirties, enjoy more energy, mental clarity (we used to be so fatigued after working hard all day, we had no energy or mind left to enjoy the time together at night), that life is—at last—a PLEASURE." No bureaucrat, she wrote, had the right to take all this away; "I demand to remain free in my choice to supplement my diet any way I please without your interference."[28] Other consumers answered the FDA with stronger language. "How in the hell will making me get a prescription to buy a harmless one-hundred milligram ascorbic acid tablet preserve my free choice?" asked one writer from Blue Ridge, Georgia.[29] For consumers, unless and until the FDA could document harm, they demanded the right to purchase what they wanted. Aspirin, cough medicines, and other products are potentially dangerous; why not restrict purchase of them? "Until you do, I feel you are being discriminatory and grossly unfair and are taking away some of my cherished rights as an American citizen," opined one woman from Roseburg, Oregon.[30] Another writer stated the consumer rights' argument succinctly: "If I want to spend my money on vitamin tablets that contain 10,000 U.S.P. units that is my business, not yours, and I wish you would stick your nose out of it."[31]

The FDA and American consumers found themselves on opposite sides of an ongoing debate familiar to all regulatory agencies overseeing consumer issues and common in the consumer movement in general. At heart of the debate is the question of the limits of consumer information. How and when is it possible to give consumers sufficient information for them to make informed decisions? Under what circumstances can they evaluate advertising and therapeutic claims? At what point is the direction of an expert necessary? Will consumers make choices based on the best available information? Or will they be deceived by promotional campaigns, well-meaning but inappropriate spokespersons, and unscrupulous manufacturers? With no clear scientific consensus on vitamin supplementation, this debate became particularly acrimonious.

The actions of the FDA and much of its self-defensive publicity suggested that its officials believed the American consumer was incompetent, easily and unthinkingly swayed by advertising hype. The growth in vitamin sales and the voluminous correspondence generated by the proposed regulations were evidence to the agency that the public was buying the "false hopes" of the industry. In this scenario, it was the FDA's duty and responsibility to prevent consumers from making fools of themselves. Concerned consumers interpreted the situation very differently. They could and they were making informed decisions. Whether they learned of vitamin supplementation from books and newspapers, health food stores, friends, physicians, or from advertising, they knew from personal experience that vitamin supplementation was their nutritional choice. Most of them granted the FDA the authority to protect them from harmful products, but strenuously objected when the agency arrogantly sought to place vitamins in this category. After all, these consumers knew vitamin supplements were healthful and not harmful. It is important to note that these consumers saw themselves as the very informed citizenry the FDA promoted. They had considered their options, and their information and experience led them to a conclusion that differed dramatically from the FDA's.

The agency believed that the scientific and medical bases for consumers' arguments were weak or nonexistent. Moreover, the FDA's files are filled with consumer correspondence advocating a vast range of questionable health practices. To the FDA, the support for vitamin supplementation was another example of American consumers buying into a fraudulent health claim based on spurious science, much the same as the controversy over laetrile and other cancer treatments outside of standard medical practice. Therefore, agency officials did not recognize the significance of this correspondence. However, the sheer volume of the public response should have alerted them to the power of the vitamin-taking consumer.

Public airing of scientific disagreements gave consumers a handle on the controversy, a handle they used to evaluate the role of vitamins in their own lives. The FDA set itself up as the arbiter of the scientific evidence and the judge of what was healthful, concluding that there was insufficient evidence to support vitamin supplementation. Consumers considered the same data and concluded otherwise. They integrated elements of the scientific debate with their personal and familial experiences and determined that vitamins were vital to their health and well-being. Convinced of the importance of vitamins, consumers tried to persuade the FDA, but to no avail. Though the agency, secure in its own beliefs, gave vitamin-taking consumers little satisfaction, Congress was more willing to listen to the public's concerns about "health freedom."

# CHAPTER 8

# "Intensity" Makes the Difference

## Vitamins in the Political Process

Consumers' voices were heard not only in the offices of the Food and Drug Administration. They were also heard in the halls of the legislature where they joined with the voices of members of Congress in protest over vitamin regulations. It was in the Congress and in the courts that the FDA's efforts met the most effective resistance. For nearly a decade, from the late 1960s into the mid-1970s, Congress struggled with the problem of where to draw the line between governmental regulation and the individual's right to choose. At the same time, vitamin manufacturers and health-food store owners initiated suits challenging the agency's power. Both the judicial system and the legislative system, in effect, debated the appropriate function of scientific experts and the limits of scientific authority. By 1976, the Proxmire Amendment denied the FDA the role the agency had claimed. With reasons based on consumer's rights and contemporary science, lawmakers prohibited the FDA from regulating vitamin products.

Initially Congress sought to curb the FDA's authority over vitamins in the late 1960s. The first bill, commonly known as H.R. 643, was introduced by California congressman Craig Hosmer, whose district included the offices of the National Health Federation. Other representatives quickly supported Hosmer's legislation.[1] By 1973, the bill had attracted over 206 co-sponsors, drawn from an extremely wide political range. Hosmer, to quote commentator Nicholas von Hoffman, was "the right-wing Republican who once suggested that we could scare the North Vietnamese into surrendering if the Air Force would only drop, not tac nukes, but voodoo dolls on our enemy." On the other end of the cosponsors' spectrum was Congresswoman Bella Abzug, Democrat from New York, who, in von Hoffman's phrase, "wears her broad brim hats pulled way down over her left eye." Such diverse legislators joined in sponsoring the bill because of pressure from their constituents, consumers convinced that the FDA was trying to take away the vitamins they needed for their good health. Reportedly by the early 1970s, more constituents expressed opinions on this subject than on any other issue except the Vietnam War.[2]

In 1973, House hearings on Hosmer's bill showcased the concerns of House members and forced the FDA further into a defensive posture. Under the bill, the FDA would be prohibited from limiting the potency, number, combination, amount, or variety of vitamins in products unless the agency could prove that the product was "intrinsically injurious to health." The FDA could not designate which combinations and potencies could be sold. Moreover, the agency could require warning labels only on products proven "intrinsically injurious to health." Basically the bill continued the FDA's traditional role of consumer protector while it restricted broadening the agency's mandate to products that had not been proven harmful. Though the ostensible reason for the 1973 hearings was Hosmer's bill, in reality the discussions focused almost exclusively on the FDA's proposed regulations.

The bill horrified the FDA, and several members of the agency voiced opposition at the hearings. Commissioner Schmidt claimed that passage of the bill would "promote widespread consumer fraud." He insisted that the agency's regulations were based on the "best scientific judgment available to the country at this time." He was especially worried that the wording of the bill shifted the burden of proof and safety entirely to the FDA. The agency staff was already stretched beyond its capacity; how could it handle even more? Peter Barton Hutt, assistant general counsel of the FDA, argued that the regulations were needed to prevent fraud. Ogden C. Johnson, the FDA's acting director of Nutrition and Consumer Sciences, Bureau of Foods, emphasized that there was not enough information on the chronic and possibly toxic effects of megadosing.[3] Basically, the FDA officials continued to present themselves as protectors of consumers, using science to shield the American public from nutrition fraud.

The hearings attracted numerous other speakers, including scientists, members of Congress, agents from the food-supplement industries such as the National Health Federation, National Nutritional Foods Association, and Miles Laboratories, spokespersons from health care organizations such as the American Medical Association, and delegates from large and small consumer groups such as the National Retired Teachers Association–American Association of Retired Persons, the Federation of Homemakers, and the Health Action Committee. Most of those testifying disagreed emphatically with the FDA's view of itself and its actions; most supported Hosmer's bill or a variant of it. Some of these witnesses may have been self-serving; industry representatives, for example, wanted to preserve their economic position. Some may have been, particularly in the eyes of FDA officials, sleazy; the agency often remarked that several National Health Federation officers had been convicted of health fraud.[4] Nevertheless, their testimony resonates with the concerns of a large segment of the American public. The pronouncements of the agency, on the other hand, clearly were out of step with the nutritional beliefs of many consumers. Speakers at the House hearings repeated arguments made popular in the press and found over and over in letters to the FDA; most frequently they focused on consumers' rights and the arrogance of the FDA.

Some supporters of the agency's position did appear at the hearings. Several researchers, from both academia and industry, contended that the FDA regulations were based on "sound scientific evidence and are clearly in the public interest." For instance, they supported the agency's contention that there was no evidence for the effectiveness of vitamin intake in excess of 150 percent RDA.[5] These scientists included employees of Miles Laboratories, who obviously found that the 1973 version of the

FDA regulations no longer threatened them. Specializing in daily supplements such as One-A-Day, rather than super high-potency products, Miles would have little trouble complying with the proposed rules, which could also eliminate some of their less cautious competitors. Other scientists stressed that the proposals were needed for consumer protection. Charles N. Jolly of Miles Laboratories explained that the regulations were needed to simplify the market. At present there were too many products available, the market being too confusing for the average consumer to judge vitamin products.[6] This need for consumer protection was echoed by William R. Roy, congressman from Kansas and member of the hearing committee. "I practiced medicine for 15 years," he remembered, and "I have seen more people come in with more jugs of more things that were absolutely useless which they had received from their local naturopath or others who we presume were practicing the healing arts."[7] In general, though, proponents of the FDA's proposed regulations were in short supply at the hearings.

The vast majority of speakers made it clear that they objected to the FDA and its regulations. Many of these witnesses were members of Congress who invariably opened their remarks with a statement about the incredible amount of mail they had received and how constituents were incensed with the FDA's actions. Whether they personally advocated vitamin supplementation or not, the legislators were being told by voters in their districts to curb the FDA. At any rate, the motivations of individual members of Congress are less significant than the impact of vast numbers of them speaking against the FDA on behalf of their constituents.

Numerous witnesses questioned the scientific basis of the FDA regulations, bringing the scientific controversy into the political process. Some claimed that "new discoveries are being made every day regarding the therapeutic advantages of high vitamin intake."[8] Others reminded committee members that scientists themselves did not agree on the use of RDAs as nutritional standards. Moreover, the RDAs were not all that the FDA promoted them to be. One witness characterized them as "guesswork."[9] Another, an esteemed vitamin researcher named Roger J. Williams, critiqued how RDAs were developed by the Food and Nutrition Board. He told the committee that members of the board "merely get together, and from the information available, they do the best they can in setting up what they think would be safe and desirable values." His opinion of RDAs differed profoundly from that of the FDA: "I look upon these values in a very different light from something that came down from the mountain by Moses."[10]

Other arguments at the hearings were more medically oriented. Innumerable speakers denied that the American diet was nutritionally sound. They discussed studies documenting the poor nutrition of various groups within the country. Moreover, they pointed out that consumers would not be helped if vitamins were transformed into prescription drugs. (In discussing vitamin supplementation, witnesses rarely spoke of the FDA's three separate categories. They concentrated their comments almost exclusively on those classified as drugs, which they believed would make vitamins into prescription-only items.) Physicians, many witnesses declared, did not have sufficient nutrition education. Ruth Desmond, president of the Federation of Homemakers, a national consumer group, was particularly concerned about this issue. Ordinarily the federation supported the work of the FDA, she explained, but for the first time the organization found itself in disagreement with the agency because "busy physicians, who receive *virtually no training* in medical schools, by their own admission, will not detect their patients' special requirements for larger amounts of certain vitamins."[11] Doctors not only lacked knowledge, many were downright hostile. The American Medical Association consistently supported FDA regulations and numerous physicians publicly opposed megadosing. Obviously, doctors did not always share consumers' faith in vitamin supplementation.

Witnesses also addressed the question of costs resulting from the regulations. One representative estimated that vitamin costs could rise as much as four or five times current prices.[12] The hearings provided a platform for public testimonials on the role of vitamin supplementation in the American diet and the role of the FDA in protecting the public's economic, as well as physical, well-being. Clearly few speakers anticipated consumers rejecting vitamin supplementation. They assumed that people would continue to take vitamins, but that under the regulations they would cost more, either through prescriptions or in quantity.

The principal argument explored at the hearings revolved around the charge that the FDA regulations were a needless infringement on consumers' rights.[13] To many, consumer protection was an important aspect of the FDA's regulatory role, but the agency was reaching beyond its authority. As Wendell Wyatt, congressman from Oregon, analyzed the situation, the agency was shifting roles. In attempting to expand its control of dangerous and unsafe drugs, it was now encompassing items "as innocuous and potentially beneficial as supplemental vitamins and minerals. . . . The protector has become the antagonist."[14] Evidently, for many speakers, the limits of scientific knowledge did not require the FDA's intercession, as the the agency claimed. Rather, the lack of definitive research left space for consumers to make their own decisions, for consumers' right to choose.

Other speakers considered the problem one of the imposition of a nutritional philosophy. As John A. Blatnik, congressman from Minnesota, characterized the situation; the FDA focused on "sickness" and "cure"; it saw vitamins as therapies for illness. The health-food industry saw vitamins as "an investment in optimal health." The congressman, maintaining that consumers had the right to choose between the "diametrically opposed" views of vitamins, declared, "I do not see how the FDA can claim the right to impose its philosophy of nutrition on those who have subscribed to a different one."[15] Blatnik's evaluation fits with assertions by Linus Pauling and others that the FDA was using RDAs inappropriately. RDAs were designed to set the minimum needed to prevent deficiency diseases; Pauling's oft-stated goal was to establish a recommended level to insure optimal health, a very different perspective.[16] These contrasting views of vitamin supplements received much comment at the hearings. Most regarded the FDA's unwillingness to look beyond gross vitamin deficiencies as wrong-headed.

Consumers appearing at the hearings explicitly rejected the FDA's assumption that they were unable to evaluate nutritional evidence; they presented themselves as knowledgeable, aware buyers. People who had never thought to appear at a congressional hearing felt impelled to speak out. For example, Mrs. Lee Aikin, co-chair of the Health Action Committee, appeared nervous at the hearings and told the committee members that she was unaccustomed to speaking before Congress. She went on to describe her small group as "people who have gotten interested in vitamins because of personal health problems. We began talking over our own experiences and finally decided that we had had such very fine results in our own experience and with our family and friends that we felt a great untapped reserve of health information was not being efficiently utilized." Members of the Health Action Committee felt comfortable with and knowledgeable about their vitamin usage. Other consumers did as well, said Aikin, who told the committee that "people are not so dumb that they will continue to buy vitamins if they don't feel any better for taking them."[17] Her picture of a thoughtful consumer who decided to take vitamins contrasted sharply with the image of a deceived customer presented by the FDA. Letters written to the agency and members of Congress and other testimony at the hearings similarly depict consumers actively involved in decision making. The specific causal connections, if any, between vitamins and good health are impossible to determine, but what is undeniable is consumers' convictions of a connection, despite the FDA's disclaimers.

For years Craig Hosmer introduced his bill to curb the powers of the FDA. Each time, despite numerous co-sponsors, his efforts failed. However, congressional adversaries were not limited to the House of Representatives; the agency faced an attack from the Senate as well. In August 1974, the upper house entered the controversy directly as it opened its own hearings into the role of the FDA in vitamin regulations. To indicate the fervor of consumers for vitamin supplementation, an aide to Senator Edward M. Kennedy of Massachusetts, chair of the subcommittee conducting the hearings, noted that the vitamin issue had brought "more mail into our mailroom recently than even Watergate."[18] The specific legislation debated by the Senate was the Proxmire Amendment, which would prohibit the FDA from regulating vitamin products. In the mid-1970s, much of the controversy between the Senate and the agency centered on Senator William Proxmire of Wisconsin. In the history of the Proxmire Amendment we can see some of the scientific, political, and personal components that shape the congressional legislative process.

For several reasons, Proxmire was predisposed to take a critical role in the legislative battle with the FDA.[19] The senator was already known for disagreeing with the agency. His 1972 publication, *Uncle Sam—Last of the Big Time Spenders*, included a scathing attack on the FDA. He described the agency as a regulatory bureaucracy riddled with conflict of interest and maintained that it typically "act[s] in the interests of the big drug companies, while routinely harassing small firms or individual innovators through the police power the FDA exercises."[20] He routinely questioned FDA actions. His resistance to the FDA's attempts to regulate vitamins was also fueled by a personal commitment to supplementation. His popular self-help book, *You Can Do It! Senator Proxmire's Exercise, Diet and Relaxation Plan*, advised the regular use of vitamins. He admitted that "the case for them is tentative" and cautioned readers to see their physician for physiological problems; yet he concluded that he takes vitamins "just to be on the safe side." His book did not recommend excessive doses of vitamins but concluded that "a limited amount, even if your diet is good, can't hurt, and it may enable you to hedge your bets in case the preponderant medical opinion of today turns out to be wrong."[21] Vitamin pills were not panaceas, but the typical American diet was not adequate and balanced. For Proxmire, as for many other American consumers, vitamin pills represented a form of nutritional insurance.

Moreover, from his earliest years in the Senate, Proxmire had been known as a consumer advocate. Proxmire went back to Wisconsin every week and on vacations; he talked with constituents and heard from small health-food store proprietors and consumers about their fears over the FDA proposed regulations. He also received letters from worried constituents. According to Howard E. Shuman, former administrative assistant to Proxmire,

• • • • • • • • • • • • • • • • • • • • • • • • • • • • • • • • • • • • • • •

the senator's office received some form letters and preprinted postcards, but more persuasive were the detailed personal letters which alerted the office to the vitamin issue. "If [constituents] get to the place where they care about [an issue], when they write a personal letter and Prox comes to town and they go to see him or they meet him at the airport, then that means they're stirred up about it. . . . If a narrow interest group doesn't make a good case, people will get tired and not be intense about it. See, intensity is what made the difference."[22] Proxmire's efforts also attracted attention from consumers beyond Wisconsin. One citizen from California seconded Proxmire's opinion of the FDA, condemning "the arrogance and impudence of FDA Commissioner Alexander M. Schmidt" and suggesting that "this man should be removed from work for government, for he believes he is bigger and greater than we the people." The writer ended by urging: "Fight, Senator, fight. Do it now. We, the people can't wait for the FDA to kill us off."[23]

Proxmire's inclinations were supported by his staff. Shuman was a pivotal player, a staffer who had previously worked with Senator Paul H. Douglas of Illinois, one of the critics of the FDA bureaucracy in the 1950s and 1960s. While in Douglas's office, Shuman had met Clinton Miller and Dr. Miles Robinson, both of the National Health Federation. In 1972, Miller visited Shuman in Proxmire's office to alert them to the FDA attempts to control vitamin products and to urge Proxmire to introduce a bill to prohibit the FDA's regulations. Miller also introduced Shuman to Milton Bass, legal representative of the vitamin-supplementation industry.

Two simple, intertwining factors underlay the push for Proxmire's bill, which were the same factors evident in the House deliberations, in consumers' letters to the agency, and in press reports. One was the ambiguity of scientific evidence; the other, the limits of governmental authority. Whether arguing for or against vitamins, proponents could cite data to support their position, data interpreted quite differently by their opponents. For Proxmire and others opposed to the FDA regulations, these scientific and medical disagreements meant that the agency did not have the scientific basis for restricting vitamin supplementation, and without scientific evidence, it did not have the authority to restrict vitamin purchases. Shuman summed up Proxmire's involvement quite simply: "It was pretty spontaneous. We had absolutely nothing to do with the health food industry. They hadn't contributed to Proxmire; he didn't take contributions. So we had no reason to take it on, except that we thought it was an important issue."[24] And take it on Proxmire did.

On 12 December 1973, Proxmire addressed the Senate chamber on the "hostility and prejudice" of the FDA. He entered into the record newspaper columns denouncing the FDA's "most autocratic, most arrogant, most infuriating" proposals, reports of scientists disagreeing with the FDA's use of RDAs, and articles documenting the low nutritional level of the American diet and the efficacy of vitamin supplementation. He asserted that the agency did not need the new authority it sought in order to protect the American consumer. It had the power to restrict toxic products; it had the power to prohibit the sale of products falsely labeled. Therefore, "so long as the vitamins or minerals are nontoxic in the quantities recommended, and provided there is accurate labeling or the absence of false labeling, the FDA should not interfere except to carry out its existing legal responsibilities to see that food is manufactured in clean circumstances, etc." The Proxmire amendment would require the FDA to preserve the status quo: "the Secretary shall not limit the potency, number, combination, amount, or variety or any synthetic or natural vitamin, mineral or other nutritional substance, or ingredient of any food for special dietary uses if the amount recommended to be consumed does not ordinarily render it injurious to health."[25]

On 10 June 1974, Proxmire again spoke before the Senate in support of legislation to prevent the FDA from implementing vitamin regulations. This time he focused on the RDAs, a bone of contention for many opponents of the FDA rules. RDAs were established by the Food and Nutrition Board of the National Research Council; Proxmire considered its scientific objectivity compromised, accusing board members of "unconscionable conflict of interest." As proof, the senator pointed out that there were

• • • • • • • • • • • • • • • • • • • • • • • • • • • • • • • • • •

many connections between the board and industry: scientists on the board held academic positions supported by industry money; they appeared as witnesses on behalf of pharmaceutical and food manufacturers; and their research was funded from federal and private grants. Given the realities of funding scientific research, innumerable investigators faced similar circumstances, as the case of Harry Steenbock had demonstrated long ago. But in Proxmire's eyes, these monetary connections meant that the board's RDAs were "an arbitrary, unscientific and tainted standard." And thus, "the proposal to subject safe vitamins and minerals to regulation as drugs by the FDA if they are sold in quantities of 150 percent or more of the so-called RDA is a biased, unscientific, and capricious standard."[26] In the ensuing months, Alfred E. Harper, the chair of the Committee on Recommended Dietary Allowances of the National Academy of Sciences–National Research Council, frequently responded to Proxmire's charges against the RDAs and defended the FDA's proposals, both in the press and in correspondence. Proxmire's rejoinders repeated that the RDAs were "based on the conflicts of interest and self-serving views of certain portions of the food industry and their paid scientists." He even attacked Harper for being unduly influenced by General Foods, the corporation that sponsored Harper's academic chair at MIT and later at the University of Wisconsin.[27]

The senator reached an even greater audience during the Senate hearings on the Proxmire bill in August 1974. Press coverage was extensive, reporting in detail from the hearing room and liberally quoting Proxmire, Schmidt, and other principals, particularly their more graphic charges. An especially popular sound bite was Proxmire's accusation that the FDA was "trying to play God."[28]

Many of the scientists, elected officials, and consumer representatives who had appeared at the House hearings returned to the Capitol for the Senate proceedings, repeating arguments heard in the Hosmer hearings. Proxmire also repeated many of his earlier arguments, including his claim that the RDAs were "arbitrary and subjective and capricious."[29] Moreover, he noted the poor dietary habits of the American populace and warned that the regulations would force up vitamin prices, push small health-food stores out of business, and would leave the market controlled by "big-wigs" such as Miles One-A-Day, which would lead to less competition in the vitamin field.[30]

Some of the witnesses at the Senate hearings spoke against the Proxmire bill. Scientist-supporters backed the FDA and explained that the RDAs were not capricious. They worried that vitamin supplementation gave people a false sense of security and thus caused them to bypass their doctors when they needed medical attention.[31] Commissioner Schmidt feared that the Proxmire bill would encourage nutrition fraud. He pointed out that current regulations demanded that problems be handled on a case-by-case basis, a procedure so time-consuming and expensive that the agency could not efficiently handle fraudulent products. The FDA needed these new rules to protect consumers more effectively.[32] Dr. Victor Herbert went further, claiming that Proxmire's legislation would promote health quackery and "castrate the FDA in the field of human nutrition."[33] According to Herbert, the regulations were needed for consumer safety; Proxmire's legislation would "allow any nutrition quack to sell as much of any vitamin as he chooses, regardless of toxicity." Proxmire replied sharply; "That's absolutely false." He contended that if a vitamin level of a product were toxic, the FDA already had the authority to regulate it. He was particularly upset at Herbert's use of words: the "reference to 'castrating the FDA in the vitamin field,'" he declared, "implies that we are trying to take away some of the FDA's present power in this area and that's false too because our bill does not change existing law in any way."[34]

As in other forums that debated the merits of the FDA proposals, the Senate hearings provided a stage for competing views of science. Some scientists insisted that there was a consensus on RDAs and their significance in human nutrition; others just as vehemently insisted on the confusion among scientific experts. Given the controversy within the scientific community, it is interesting to note that M. Daniel Tatkon, author of *The Great Vitamin Hoax* (1968), seemed unaware of the irony when he cautioned: "This committee and the Congress should not be swayed by the great names, credentials and affiliations which have been paraded before this subcommittee to give testament to the holy vitamin."[35] Tatkon was confident about which claims and which researchers he believed. But others were equally certain and they believed different scientists. Each side, pro and con, could call upon nutritionists and physicians with impressive credentials.

While consumers were engulfing the FDA with letters of protest and the House and Senate were holding hearings on the Hosmer and Proxmire legislation, manufacturers and other industry groups pursued the agency in the courts. In August 1974, during the Senate hearings, the U.S. Court of Appeals issued a decision postponing enforcement of the vitamin regulations. Judge Henry J. Friendly agreed that the FDA had presented an impressive case for reform to halt extravagant claims on the part of the vitamin industry, and he insisted that he was "broadly sustaining the regulations." The general counsel of the National Nutritional Foods Association, Milton Bass, characterized the ruling as a "mixed bag with something for everybody." Contrary to Bass's analysis and the judge's claim, however, the court's decision in effect stymied the most significant aspect of the proposals. In particular, the court ruled that the FDA could not automatically classify products containing more than 150 percent of RDA as drugs. In February 1975, the Supreme Court let stand the lower court's ruling.[36] These judicial decisions, the House and Senate hearings, and the extensive correspondence from troubled consumers forced the FDA to rethink its regulations.

Neither the House hearings of 1973 nor the Senate hearings of 1974 resulted in passage of legislation. Neither did the FDA successfully implement its regulations. But with the threat of congressional action and the court decisions limiting the agency's authority, the FDA rewrote the regulations and issued new proposals in 1975. Under these, the agency would treat most vitamin products as food, not drugs. Schmidt stated, "We believe the revised regulations are a substantial improvement over the original approach because they will be less subject to misinterpretation and misrepresentation." They would provide consumers with "more and better information upon which to make their purchasing decisions."[37] The new proposals would regulate vitamins as food and would control for safety only. Thus a product containing more than 150 percent of the RDA could be sold without proof of efficacy. Vitamin C products, for instance, could be marketed in any potency.[38]

Some supporters of earlier FDA proposals were quick to criticize the more lenient rules. The Health Research Group, a staunch advocate of greater control of vitamins, accused the FDA of backing down under pressure from the health-food industry, pointing out that the new proposals shifted the burden of proof from industry to the FDA, a burden that the agency was in no position to shoulder. If vitamins were classified as drugs, then manufacturers were required to demonstrate efficacy and safety; if classified as food, the FDA itself would need to conduct the tests for efficacy and safety, but the agency lacked the resources to do so.[39] If the revisions did not satisfy former proponents, neither did they please those who had fought the agency for years. Despite the revisions defining vitamins as foods, many feared that the agency still hoped to restrict vitamin supplementation. The FDA had created an avalanche of opposition that could not be stopped or even deflected by revision.

Letters continued to flow to Congress and into the agency, the lawyers continued to prepare their court appeals, and Proxmire continued to push for passage of his legislation.[40] In September 1974, Proxmire's bill was approved by a vote of eighty-one to ten as an amendment to the Health Professions Educational Assistance Act, but it died in committee when House and Senate conferees could not agree on its terms. In February 1975, Proxmire reintroduced legislation to prohibit the FDA from controlling vitamins as drugs, declaring, "Since the FDA first proposed their regulations in June of 1966 a Damoclean sword has been hanging over the heads of the vitamin consumer, the small health food stores, and the vitamin producers in the form of these unnecessary and arbitrary requirements."[41] The bill passed through a series of revisions in consultation with House and Senate representatives. As Proxmire persisted, he reiterated in Congress and in the press that vitamins were not drugs and should not be classified as drugs. If they were defined by the FDA as drugs, then the agency could require the manufacturer to provide proof that they were both safe and effective. "But," the senator noted, "the FDA has already proclaimed its view—time and time again—that vitamins in excess of RDAs are NOT efficacious. There [is] no way the vitamin people could win against a stacked deck like the FDA."[42] In a debate over conflicting interpretations of scientific evidence, the view of the agency in power would carry the day. Basically each case would be a replay of the Acnotabs experience: the manufacturer needed to supply evidence, but the FDA would be the judge of that evidence, and the agency had already declared that there was not sufficient evidence.

On 11 December 1975, the Senate passed the National Heart and Lung Institutes Bill, which was identical to the House version except for the addition of the Proxmire Amendment to prohibit the FDA from regulating vitamins. This difference sent the bills to a conference committee. It took much negotiating between House and Senate staff members to achieve a compromise that would pass both houses. Shuman, who was intimately involved in these deliberations, remembers that the House staff was supportive of the FDA. However, the overwhelming Senate vote of ninety to two persuaded them to compromise. On 2 April 1976, the committee agreed on a bill including the vitamin amendment. Later that month, after nearly ten years of legislative debate, both houses finally passed legislation stating that "the Secretary may not classify any natural or synthetic vitamin or mineral (or combination thereof) as a drug solely because it exceeds the level of potency which the Secretary determines is nutritionally rational or useful."[43]

For the first time in its history, Congress had restricted the powers of the FDA. In the words of historian James Harvey Young, the law represented "the first retrogressive step in federal legislation respecting self-treatment wares since enactment of the initial Food and Drugs Act in 1906."[44] Some bemoaned the Vitamin Amendment of 1976 as a significant step backward, as a setback for consumer protection; others saw it as maintaining the status quo, preventing the FDA from expanding its powers irrationally, and a triumph of consumer power.

The FDA's opinion of its defeat was clear: its concern for consumers drove it to propose regulations intended to "improve the consumer's economic protection" by limiting the marketing of irrational and useless products. With the restrictions of the new law, "it will be up to consumers to decide on their own the kinds and amounts of vitamins and minerals they need to supplement their diet, and whether massive doses of these substances are nutritionally useful or a waste of money."[45] Given the agency's views of vitamin supplementation and the consumer, clearly the FDA expected that many would waste their money. Others, however, saw the situation in a much different light. They did not believe that the only way to evaluate vitamin sufficiency was the presence or absence of gross vitamin deficiency diseases. Nor did they believe that the RDAs represented the maximum optimal levels for vitamin intake. Disagreeing with the agency, they demanded their right to vitamin supplementation. Consumers, the vitamin manufacturers, the health-food industry, and concerned members of Congress fought the FDA because they believed that the agency had neither the authority nor the scientific evidence to make these decisions for consumers.

Despite passage of the Vitamin Amendment of 1976, the controversy did not disappear. Periodically over the next several years, it resurfaced to be debated again in the pages of the popular press.[46] Recently, more attention has been focused on RDAs, their development and use. As early as 1986 popular articles describing the advantages and disadvantages of vitamin supplementation mentioned controversy within the National Academy of Sciences over the RDA revisions. Though the RDAs are scheduled to be revised every five years, in 1985 the committee overseeing the revisions disbanded before releasing a report. Evidently, outside nutrition experts disagreed strongly with the draft proposals. Moreover, some committee members wanted to lower the RDAs for vitamins A and C, an action that appeared to contradict another NAS report which stated that additional vitamins A and C in the American diet might help protect against cancer. With the release of the 1989 revisions, scientists expressed dissatisfaction with the principle underlying the RDAs. They had been established as benchmarks in the prevention of gross vitamin deficiency diseases, but those diseases are rare. The review process is very expensive, costing between $500,000 and $1 million each, and ignores suggestive though inconclusive evidence of the benefits of massive doses of some vitamins. Significantly, by the late 1980s, the revision committee conceded that RDAs are "neither minimal requirements nor necessarily optimal levels of intake." Moreover, the RDAs were established only for healthy persons; the committee did not address evidence that sick people's needs might differ. In addition, the RDA review process focused on deficiency diseases and current health status, while to other scientists the interesting and important questions had to do with the risks of cancer, heart disease, osteoporosis, and other chronic diseases in the future.[47] The same confusion over the use of scientific evidence that plagued the FDA's attempts to regulate vitamin products is reflected in the confusion over the meaning and usefulness of RDAs today.

In the 1990s we saw the development of a new legislative battle between the Food and Drug Administration and Congress over the limits of the agency's authority over vitamins. Under the 1990 Nutritional Labeling and Education Act, FDA Commissioner David Kessler attempted to establish controls over the claims manufacturers can make for vitamin products. Fearing that such action would effectively reclassify these products as drugs and would deny all but the most basic health claims, opponents once again mobilized to battle with the agency. On 13 August 1993, health-food stores throughout the country sponsored a Blackout Day. Retailers marked with black dots products they believed were threatened by Kessler's proposals, and they stretched black crepe paper over shelves of items "destined to disappear under the FDA regulations." They distributed sample letters and petitions to customers with the admonition, "Take Action for Health Freedom," and they designed eye-catching posters of dinosaurs that reflected the Hollywood hit of the season, *Jurassic Park* (Figure 8-1).[48]

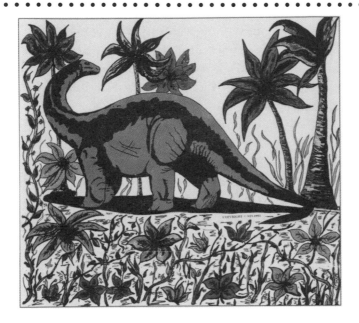

What do Dietary Supplements and Dinosaurs
Have in Common?

Nothing...YET!

Tell Congress to Keep it That Way!

Write Your Elected Representative NOW.

**Figure 8-1:** "What do Dietary Supplements and
Dinosaurs Have in Common?" 1993. (Courtesy of
Cheryl Hughes, Lancaster, Calif.)

Once again health-food stores galvanized their customers to
contact their representatives in Congress. And once again, a
broad range of members of Congress supported them. Proxmire
had retired from the Senate, but Senator Orrin G. Hatch of Utah
joined the struggle with the FDA, along with Bill Richardson, congressman from New Mexico. Liberal legislators such as Senator
Barbara Boxer of California signed on as co-sponsors of legislation to restrict the FDA's power over vitamin pills.[49] Hatch had

several reasons for defending vitamin consumers and the health food industry. From all accounts he is an avid user of vitamins, "sometimes offering visitors to his office what one source described as 'glasses of green goop.' "[50] Furthermore, vitamins are an important industry in Utah.

The Hatch-Richardson bill was aptly called the Health Freedom Act, reflecting the same concerns for the freedom of choice expressed during the battles of the 1960s and 1970s; it was intended to protect the rights of consumers. It also directly addressed the lack of scientific consensus. The FDA regulations demanded that manufacturers demonstrate "significant scientific agreement" before placing a health claim on a label or in catalogs or brochures; Hatch-Richardson allowed health claims that reflected "the totality of scientific evidence" and are "truthful and non-misleading."[51]

Senator Hatch fought for "the right of millions of Americans to products that have been used safely for millennia." He linked vitamin supplementation and the cost of health care, claiming the benefits of regular use of vitamins would lower our nation's health bill. He called on the government to encourage, not discourage, vitamin takers. In insisting that the standard of "significant scientific agreement" was too limited, Hatch pointed to the debate over folic acid. As early as 1982, studies showed that increasing the folic acid in the diets of pregnant women resulted in fewer cases of neural tube defects in their children. The Centers for Disease Control recommended the use of folic acid in 1991; the Department of Health and Human Services recommended its use in 1992. However, it was not until January 1994 that the FDA approved the claim. Hatch criticized the FDA's lag time, which suggested that the FDA's standard was too restricted. Thus, Hatch recommended holding vitamin claims to a "slightly lower standard," namely "significant scientific evidence." Otherwise, he feared, "no claims will be made, consumers will receive no information beyond what they ferret out for themselves, and health costs will continue to rise."[52]

In many respects the debate of the 1990s replays the arguments of the 1970s: who decides the validity and power of scientific evidence? Should we be governed by the FDA's definition of "significant scientific agreement" or a more fluid and less dogmatic "significant scientific evidence"? Many consumers believe that vitamin C helps prevent and even cure colds. Do they base this belief on personal experience, on "significant scientific agreement," or on "significant scientific evidence"? How far should the FDA's interpretation of scientific and medical data go in defining consumers' choices?

What is clear from the history of the FDA's attempts to control the vitamin market is that on this issue, at least, the agency is usually working against the grain of public opinion. Each time the FDA has promoted regulations, it has faced increasing resistance. The stream of correspondence that flowed to Congress in the 1960s became a torrent in the 1970s. By the 1990s, in a single twelve-month period ending in the spring of 1994, Congress received more than 100,000 letters and telephone calls in support of the Hatch-Richardson bill.[53] By May 1994, the bill had 65 co-sponsors in the Senate and 249 in the House.[54] By October 1994, yet again, Congress blocked the FDA. Under compromise legislation, the agency retains the power to approve or disapprove claims for disease prevention, such as a product's ability to fight cancer. However, the bill also allows manufacturers wide latitude to promote "structure and function" nutritional claims. That is, a product can claim that vitamin A is necessary for good vision, without fear of FDA interference.[55]

Over the decades, the FDA has equated vitamin supplementation and health quackery and has been frustrated with the need for slow and expensive case-by-case litigation when it sees instances of nutrition fraud. Consequently, it has attempted to design regulations to simplify the control of vitamin products. Confident in its stand on supplementation and convinced of its interpretation of scientific results, the agency misjudged the power of the industry, the significance of the lack of scientific consensus, and, most particularly, the extent of consumers' commitment to vitamins. The mystique and power of vitamins convinced many people that they needed dietary supplements: at minimum vitamins are useful as health insurance, while at maximum, they are required for good health. The FDA's efforts did little to inspire the confidence of vitamin takers in the 1960s and 1970s, and they have left a legacy of fear and anxiety, emotions that fueled an equally strong resistance to the agency's actions in the 1990s.

# Vitamania?

## Vitamins in Late Twentieth-Century United States

The history of vitamins is a cautionary tale. It reveals that the rhetorical power of science in our culture is incredibly potent, so potent that many people wrapped themselves in the flag of science. What is true for vitamins is repeated in many other aspects of American culture. In the past few decades we have faced questions about the dangers of radon, the risks of fluoride, the hazards of alar, and the perils of bovine growth hormones, to name just a few hot topics. Partisans of these controversies argue with contemporary science, with contradictory and contested science. Each claimant professes to be a holder of special knowledge. So it has been with vitamins.

The mystique, the magic, the allure of vitamins have fascinated people from the time the word was coined in 1912. Undeniably, the micronutrients produced miraculous cures in cases of gross deficiency diseases. These wonders inspired speculation about vitamin's other health-giving and health-preserving actions, speculation built on public announcements about the role of vitamins in human nutrition. In our consumer culture, vitamins became a symbol of the benefits of science available to all. Yet the scientific evidence remained inconsistent and in dispute. Increasingly sophisticated studies produced more questions than they answered, and we continue to debate the crucial role of vitamins in good health and the significance of vitamins for optimal well-being.

● ● ● ● ● ● ● ● ● ● ● ● ● ● ● ● ● ● ● ● ● ● ● ● ● ● ● ● ● ● ● ● ● ● ● ● ●

Over the years, scientific and health-care professionals, advertisers and manufacturers, consumer activists and government officials, all joined the fray. Regardless of whether they supported or opposed vitamin pills, regardless of their level of economic or professional self-interest in the issue, they all employed two over-arching themes to justify their involvement in this very public and contentious debate: consumer protection and the authority of science.

As early as the 1910s, when vitamins were just entering the public arena, proponents and opponents of vitamin supplementation positioned themselves as champions of consumer protection, protecting the consumer's health and the consumer's wallet. Proponents claimed that the American food supply lacked the necessary nutrients and that modern processing and storage further compromised its nutritional value. Moreover, even among those who could afford a wide variety of foodstuffs, the average American diet did not include all the foods necessary for balanced nutrition. Salvation, they asserted, lay in vitamin pills, which could compensate for these and other dietary problems. For supporters of vitamin supplementation, consumer protection meant vitamin products readily available on the open market. On the other side, opponents denied that vitamin products were needed to supplement the American diet. They dismissed the notion that the food supply did not provide sufficient micronutrients and insisted that everyone could and should get all the required vitamins in food. To them, an open market on vitamin supplements was a fraud perpetrated on the American consumer: consumer protection demanded a restricted market.

Whether arguing from a self-interested profit motive, from a concern for consumer protection, from a faith and conviction in the efficacy of vitamins, or from a combination of these beliefs, proponents and opponents of vitamin supplementation dressed themselves in the cloak of science. Of course, each group defined science somewhat differently. Some looked to carefully constructed laboratory research, supported by clearly articulated and well-formulated theories, as well as sophisticated, large-scale clinical trials with unequivocal results. For these observers, science was process. Others were more pragmatic; they were convinced by their own experiences and the personal experiences of others. Scientific evidence was observation and was even individualistic. Still others did not claim personal involvement in science, but based their beliefs and practices on the authority of science.

Journalists and manufacturers helped explain to the American public the secret of vitamins and what lack of these micronutrients would do to the human body. They took their argument for regular vitamin supplementation to generally well-nourished middle-class Americans. Those convinced of the importance of vitamin pills for human health and happiness fought against the skepticism and derision of those convinced that the American diet was more than sufficient to provide what was needed. Opponents of supplemental vitamins frequently declared the promoters of vitamin pills frauds and fakes, out to make a quick buck from gullible consumers. Yet more and more research studies throughout the century suggested or documented the benefits of vitamin usage for widely varying conditions in significantly different situations; and the sales of vitamin products increased.

Druggists, who stood to profit from vitamin sales, were confident that they had identified the reasons people were buying vitamin supplements. They identified the influence of wartime experiences, as well as their own well-directed promotions as the salient factors. Pharmacists maintained that World War II introduced many people to the benefits of supplementation. Workers who were given pills at their factories convinced family and friends to take them as well. Soldiers who received vitamins regularly in the service tended to continue the habit when they returned to civilian life.[1] Druggists actively encouraged vitamin sales as well. They frequently discussed the most appropriate and lucrative placement of supplements. Some stacked vitamin products behind the soda fountain where they would attract the attention of customers; clerks would then distribute free samples.[2] To introduce the younger generation to vitamins, pharmacists designed promotional campaigns particularly attractive to children. One

• • • • • • • • • • • • • • • • • • • • • • • • • • • • • • • • • • • • •

enterprising druggist distributed warm popcorn and vitamin samples to trick-or-treaters on Halloween, noting an immediate increase of 20 percent in vitamin sales.[3]

Advertising also contributed to the growth of vitamin sales.
Manufacturers fervently believed in the power of advertising to
increase the market and their own market share. Advertising ex-
penditures have increased dramatically from the late 1930s, when
Vitamins Plus was launched with a budget of $210,000. Today the
industry spends over $66 million convincing the American public
of their need for vitamin pills. Figures for drugstore promotions
are not readily available, but clearly druggists were aware of the
value of vitamin advertising and they themselves correlated increased sales with targeted promotions.

Factors outside the drugstore and industry advertising also
helped persuade people to buy vitamin pills. Pregnant women
were frequently told they needed additional micronutrients, to
protect their own health and that of their offspring. Dieters, it was
feared, in attempting to lose weight, neglected the nutritional
needs of their bodies. Certain aspects of lifestyle, such as smoking,
drinking, athletics, and vegetarianism, were believed to compromise a person's nutrition and increase the body's demand for vitamins. While accepting that the diet should provide all the
required nutrients, articles in the popular press often observed
that American diets did not. Explained one writer in *McCall's* in
1979: "The problem is that many people don't eat the right foods
because they are more fattening, more trouble and more expensive. At least those are the excuses. And it does take extra time to
assure you are getting a balanced diet." If you were one of the
many who did not, then "it makes sense to take daily multiple-
vitamin supplements to keep yourself in good health."[4] National
nutritional surveys conducted in the late 1980s increased anxiety
over the status of the average American diet. In one oft-cited survey, researchers concluded that on the day of the study, 45 percent of the population had no servings of fruit or juice and 22
percent had no vegetables. These figures demonstrated that many
Americans were not enjoying an appropriately balanced diet. At a
time when recommendations for a healthful diet included three

or more servings of vegetables a day and two or more servings of fruit, only 27 percent consumed sufficient vegetables, 29 percent sufficient fruits, and only 9 percent both fruits and vegetables. Another survey found that at least 20 percent of the U.S. population was getting less than the recommended daily allowances of vitamins A, C, $B_1$, $B_2$, and $B_6$, among other micronutrients. When journal articles in the popular press repeated statistics such as these, they implied and often flatly stated that Americans needed vitamin supplements simply to achieve the recommended daily allowances designed to avoid gross vitamin deficiency conditions.[5]

But vitamins could do more. For decades, Americans had heard that vitamins enhanced one's vitality. Early on druggists' promotions considered this a significant stimulus for growing vitamin sales. Applauding the marketing of vitamin capsules in the late 1930s, one observer remarked: "An imposing literature is arising to confirm clinical opinion that so much "below par," so-so health may frequently be due to unsubstantial quantities of vitamins. . . . Concentrates of *all* the clinically established vitamins to supplement the daily menus, and not dietary changes, are best to achieve optimal intake of vitamins and the buoyant health which they can bring about.[6] Officials of the Food and Drug Administration, physicians, and other detractors consistently maintained that vitamins did not add "pep" and "energy." But proponents of vitamin supplementation just as consistently described the invigorating effects of vitamins. Paul de Kruif, popular science writer, even advised that taking vitamins would "help stretch out your span of productive vitality."[7]

This line of reasoning was not restricted to the popular press, but spread to other forms of popular culture as well. It was even depicted in Hollywood films. For example, in *Operation Petticoat* (1959), a troubled nurse worries about the well-being of the submarine's captain. She tells the captain, "I hope you won't mind a little professional advice. But when a person is nervous and irritable, you can be sure there is something he is not getting enough of." The captain looks at her quizzically, startled by the innuendo of the statement. The nurse then continues: "Vitamins and minerals. With proper nutritional balance, you wouldn't have any gray hair at all." She informs the captain that she too used to be run-down and had a poor appetite, but now she takes vitamin pills.[8] The connection between tiredness and lack of vitamins remains a recurrent theme in popular culture, even appearing in comic strips. In the popular cartoon "Sally Forth," Sally's husband notes that she seems tired all the time and asks if it could be a vitamin deficiency. She replies that it is not a vitamin deficiency, but "some sort of help-around-the-house deficiency."[9]

According to messages in the popular press and in popular culture, either insufficient diet or lack of pep could signal the need for supplementation. And many were advising a daily vitamin even in the absence of such indications. The recommendation to take vitamins as nutritional insurance has had a long history. By the 1980s and 1990s this suggestion appeared more and more frequently, featured in the mainstream press as well as in the tabloids and from the more radical nutritionists. The authors of *Vitamin Power* (1987) believed that in order to construct a healthful diet, "meals must be strategically planned and prepared, using the very freshest, most carefully grown ingredients." Unfortunately, they believed, "this kind of labor- and time-intensive approach to nutrition is rarely feasible for the way most of us live and work."[10] Clearly the solution in late twentieth-century America was supplementation. As the results of more and more research studies became widely known, tabloid headlines such as "Super Vitamin 'A' Diet: Fight Heart Disease, Cancer . . . and Lose Weight!—Say Medical Experts" appeared with increasing regularity.[11]

But many other, less zealous writers also promoted the use of vitamin pills. The voices that counseled against vitamin supplementation, insisting that it was unnecessary and a waste of money, were increasingly drowned out by those touting the benefits of vitamins. In the 1990s, newspaper headlines such as "Vitamins Win Support as Potent Agents of Health" and "Vitamins as Life Savers" became commonplace.[12] An article in *Time* in April 1992 was typical. The author differentiated between the claims of "researchers" and those of "hard-core vitamin enthusiasts." While she gave little credence to the latter, she did remind readers that contemporary studies suggested that vitamins "play a much more complex role in assuring vitality and optimal health than was previously thought." Vitamins were discussed as preventatives against "birth defects and cataracts," against "heart disease and cancer," even potentially against "the normal ravages of aging." Since Americans did not regularly consume the recommended levels of fruits and vegetables to achieve optimal vitamin intake, the author concluded, "popping pills is a good insurance policy."[13] This line of reasoning is repeated over and over again in popular magazines such as *Ladies' Home Journal, McCall's, Glamour,* and *Newsweek,* and in daily newspapers such as the *New York Times* and the *Chicago Tribune.*[14] Articles usually cite statistics documenting that the average American's food intake provides insufficient vitamins; they discuss research demonstrating the benefits of vitamins in preventing a wide range of diseases and conditions and describe physicians who both recommend vitamins for others and take them for their own health. By 1995, dietary supplementation had become so acceptable that less radical nutrition publications such as *Nutrition Action* (published by the Center for Science in the Public Interest) advised: "Take a multivitamin for insurance," and the *Tufts University Diet and Nutrition Letter* did not even question the practice.[15]

Similarly, physicians increasingly recommended vitamin pills. Though the American Medical Association consistently maintained that healthy adults can eat an adequate diet and do not need supplements, the split among physicians over the issue widened. Evidently, in the late twentieth century "the medical community is no longer speaking with one voice."[16] In a far cry from their earlier admonishments to ignore vitamin pills, numerous physicians publicly admitted they took vitamins, and not only to ward off gross vitamin deficiency conditions. Typical was Jerome Cohen, a professor of internal medicine at the St. Louis University School of Medicine. He used to reject the idea that healthy adults needed supplemental vitamins, but a 7 June 1993 article in *Newsweek* described his current regime: "In an effort to keep his heart healthy, Cohen now starts the day with 400 international units of vitamin E—roughly the amount he would get in 25 cups of peanuts. Though he isn't sure the new regimen will do him any good, he's now happy to wager a couple of bucks a month on it."[17] These and other examples in the popular press documented the faith that medical practitioners and researchers now had in vitamin supplementation. While they were not always sure about the effectiveness of vitamin pills, they did openly confess and even promoted their personal vitamin practices.

Not content to prescribe at a distance by example, physicians prepared brochures to distribute directly to their patients. One such example, entitled "Facts about Vitamin-Mineral Supplements," listed circumstances that would make the patient "a good candidate for a vitamin-mineral supplement." "Life style factors" like smoking, drinking, and low-calorie consumption warranted the use of vitamin pills. Inadequate diet was another significant indicator, particularly "if you don't think it is possible to work on changing an inadequate diet at this time or there are too many changes to make at once."[18] No longer were physicians flatly condemning the use of vitamin pills, demanding that patients revamp their daily menus to include all the needed micronutrients. By the 1990s, vitamin supplementation was becoming a more common medical recommendation.

Throughout the 1980s and 1990s, the belief in the potential value of vitamin supplementation for optimal health and well-being and for the prevention of various diseases grew, but what was still lacking was substantial evidence based on a well-respected, large, controlled clinical trial. In this atmosphere of optimism and with a growing consensus for supplementation, the spring 1994 announcement of preliminary findings from just such a study fell like a bombshell, a bombshell that was quickly reported in publications as diverse as the *New York Times*, *Newsweek*, and *Glamour*.[19] The study of more than 29,000 male smokers in Finland was designed to test the power of the so-called antioxidants, namely, vitamin E and beta-carotene (a substance that is partly converted in the body to vitamin A). Previous research had led investigators to believe that beta-carotene lowered the risk of lung cancer. Unexpectedly, about six years into the Finnish study,

results showed that those who took beta-carotene had an 18 percent greater incidence of lung cancer than those who did not. It
appeared that supplementation increased, rather than decreased,
the chance of cancer. These shocking results led researchers to
question if people should be told to stop taking beta-carotene.

Some groups that had previously advocated beta-carotene supplementation did reverse their position, as did some individual
researchers. Others dismissed the study as flawed. Articles in the
popular media followed the debate and their presentations
brought home to the public how difficult it is to construct a mean-
ingful research project on the value of micronutrients for optimal
health. For example, the men studied had smoked for an average
of thirty-six years. Thus, it was claimed, the study showed that
beta-carotene did nothing to prevent lung cancer in people
whose lungs were already probably damaged; they may have had
subclinical cancer before the test began. The study had not been
intended to test the ability of beta-carotene to cure cancer, but
rather to prevent it. To do that, we need to study a population
that does not have a long smoking history. Not only did the men
smoke, they also tended to be overweight and to consume high-fat
diets. Therefore, many researchers claimed, we still need a study
to test how the micronutrient affects people with healthier life-
styles. Other researchers maintained that one study does not
prove anything. Moreover, judging the amount of beta-carotene
in the study, commentators concluded it was difficult to believe
that the substance was harmful. As Julie Buring, a Harvard researcher currently involved in similar studies, remarked, "The
idea that the equivalent of seven or eight carrots a day [the
amount of beta-carotene used in the study] causes cancer just
doesn't hang biologically."[20]

The controversy over the Finnish study displays how significantly our view of vitamin supplementation has shifted over the
last few decades. Articles routinely noted that many, if not most,
Americans had diets deficient in vitamins. They commonly reviewed supplementation and considered it an acceptable, widely
practiced regime, though they did not necessarily recommend

• • • • • • • • • • • • • • • • • • • • • • • • • • • • • • • • • • • •

everyone take a daily vitamin pill. An analysis of the articles on vitamin supplementation appearing in one magazine illuminates this significant shift in perspective.

The articles in *Consumer Reports* (*CR*), a publication of the consumer advocacy organization Consumers Union, are carefully researched works that represent mainstream medical consensus. They are written in consultation with medical advisors and editors, and, as with all *CR* articles, are intended to aid consumers in the market. In the mid-1980s, the magazine published a report entitled "The Vitamin Pushers," attacking the industry for overselling vitamins.[21] The thrust of this essay marked a continuation of concerns reported earlier in *CR*, a point recognized by internal CU reviewers. As one remarked on a working copy of the manuscript: "CU's failure to persuade the world (or our need to repeat this story every few years) speaks to the power of the pro-vitamin forces."[22] On later galleys of the article, an editor noted, "This story still would not convince vitamin-niks to stop." A knowing colleague added, "True—but nothing will convince the true believers."[23]

Yet acknowledging that many subscribers did take supplements, an early draft of the article had included buying suggestions: "If you still opt for supplementation, shop around for the lowest-priced multivitamin that contains no more than the RDA for any ingredients. Such pills should cost less than a nickel a day." Clearly there was disagreement on the staff because, as one editor noted in the margin, "We give people what amounts to freedom of choice ('if you opt for supplementation . . .') which to me is out of step with a story about the overselling of vitamins. I think we should be more pointed and more forceful in our advice to readers." Over the next several drafts, the sentence was changed to "If you need extra vitamins, look for the lowest-priced multivitamin that contains no more than the U.S. RDA for any ingredient. Such pills should cost less than a nickel a day." And then to: "Never take more than the RDA amounts except on medical advice." And finally to: "As a rule, don't take more than the RDA amounts except on medical advice."[24] The evolution of the article mirrored the ongoing debates in the medical and scientific communities and in the popular press. In the end, the editors of *CR* took a definite stand that painted a very negative picture of vitamin supplementation, except under the direction of a physician.

Some readers of *CR* quickly expressed their dissatisfaction with the article. Letter writers were "disappointed" and "felt let-down" by Consumers Union, which, they insisted, needed to do more research. J.W.E. wrote that the article was "a poorly researched, and extremely opinionated attack on the importance of vitamins and minerals to the health of the human. Considerable scientific and established biomedical research data was ignored, or never reviewed. I had expected considerably greater things from CU."[25] M.T. accused Consumers Union of buckling under pressure from the organized medical profession: "I am very upset when I see an article like this, because I believe that you don't know what the hell you are talking about! Consumer's Guide is famous for listening to the public—it's [*sic*] subscribers. Except when it comes to the most powerful union of all—the AMA. Then you turn your back on the people you are sworn to uphold."[26] Frequently correspondents cited personal experiences to counterbalance the article. Typical was the story told by H.R.P., who had developed recurring prostate infections, despite eating a well-balanced diet and keeping physically fit. Urologists suggested that he take vitamins to build up his immune system. After reading the available literature he agreed. Now, twelve years on this regimen had convinced him of the benefits of vitamin supplementation. As long as he continued to take his vitamins regularly, he had no problem with prostate infections and also had fewer colds. If, however, he stopped the vitamins, in about three months the infections returned. "There is no other explanation for my improved resistance to infections other than the vitamins," he concluded.[27]

Six years later, in 1992, *CR* published an article entitled "Can You Live Longer?"[28] A sidebar, "The Supplement Story: Can Vitamins Help?" demonstrated that the *CR* staff had become less rigid about vitamin supplementation.[29] The article opened with the observation that the surgeon general, the National Research Council, and the U.S. Department of Health and Human Services continued to maintain that "a balanced diet provides all the nutrients needed for good health." Next to this sentence on a draft copy of the text, one of the reviewers added that this was also Consumers Union's position. Another reviewer had a different perspective: "No—our position is more complex. We agree a balanced diet provides all necessary nutrients, but also think most Americans aren't on a balanced diet—And many would have to undertake major dietary changes to achieve balance."[30] The published sidebar suggested a decreasing animosity to vitamins as well. While CU's medical consultants would not recommend supplements for the general population, still the text explained that "while few [scientists] go so far as to make public recommendations, they freely admit that popping pills has become part of their own daily routine."[31] This 1992 piece reflected the shift occurring in many other areas of the media. Though mainstream writers did not unabashedly embrace supplementation, neither did they unilaterally debunk it.

*CR*'s most recent article, "Taking Vitamins: Can They Prevent Disease?" presented the question in a different light, one that reflected the tensions of the mid-1990s.[32] Rather than simply noting the lack of scientific consensus, the text laid out the problems and contradictions inherent in clinical trials, detailing how complex and difficult it was to evaluate the effects of micronutrients on health. For example, the article teased out various confounding factors in the Finnish study and found that it "could turn out to be a watershed. . . . But the Finnish results also could be a statistical fluke. Either way, the study makes it more important than ever for consumers to understand the science of supplementation."[33]

Unlike previous *CR* discussions of vitamin supplementation, which focused on research findings, "Taking Vitamins" concentrated on analyzing the process of research and the need for consumers to evaluate research findings carefully. Although it allowed that "millions of people with subtle deficiencies might benefit from taking a daily multivitamin/mineral supplements," it did not advocate vitamin supplementation. However, the next article in the issue, "Buying Vitamins: What's Worth the Price?" reported on the testing of eighty-six different supplements.[34] This evaluation of vitamin products was an acknowledgment that vitamin supplementation remains a major consumer area extremely popular in the United States.

Why are vitamin products so accepted? Why do people take vitamin pills? Who were and are the people buying all these products? Are they credulous dupes taken in by the fancy claims of manufacturers and by self-styled but ill-educated experts, as the Food and Drug Administration officials portrayed them? Are they concerned consumers carefully weighing the scientific evidence and opting for the comfort of "nutritional insurance"? Or are they people who devoutly believe that vitamins will protect them from the ravages of modern civilization? Though the data are imprecise, we can draw with broad strokes the characteristics of vitamin users throughout the century. Some of the evidence is constructed through inference; some is based on surveys; some is anecdotal. Taken together, these sketches show us why vitamins remain a hot issue in American society.

Letters written to the FDA, Congress, and the Consumers Union have given us some indication of consumers' rationales for supplementation. We can extract other data from marketing surveys conducted by magazines, trade associations, and manufacturers interested in increasing sales. There were a few statistical studies developed for federal agencies. Both the descriptive surveys and statistical data and the self-descriptions of vitamin users who felt threatened by pending legislation and negative magazine articles help sketch a portrait of those who believe in vitamin supplementation. From this evidence, it is abundantly clear that consumers' reactions reflect the material that appeared over and over again in the press and in promotional campaigns.

One of the earliest attempts to understand why people do, or do not, buy vitamin products was produced on behalf of Miles Laboratories. In 1953, in order to determine the most effective motivational appeals for One-A-Day advertising, the "trained psychologists" on the staff of the Institute for Research in Mass Motivations conducted over 150 interviews.[35] Though most of the people interviewed did not take vitamins regularly, they believed that the American diet was deficient. Generally, respondents agreed that vitamins are lost in storage, processing, and the prep-

aration of food, and that poor soil decreases the amount of vitamins found in vegetables and fruits. Their remarks mirrored contemporary press reports. Several people expressed faith in the
invigorating capacity of vitamin pills, another common element
in the media and advertising. "I think it helps to give you energy
and pep," the report quoted one interviewee. Another explained:
"They gave me an appetite. They say it helps your appetite and
makes you gain weight." Though this study was extremely limited,
comments such as these are useful in suggesting the depth of
vitamin knowledge among consumers.

A few years later, a larger study was conducted by *Good Housekeeping*, which surveyed 1,764 subscribers.[36] Eighty-one percent of
the households of this admittedly select group of consumers took
vitamins, and 62 percent had been using vitamins for five or more
years. Thirty-four percent of the correspondents used vitamins to
supplement their diets; 29 percent took vitamins to resist or prevent colds; 21 percent on doctors' advice; 17 percent to maintain
general health; and 16 percent for increased energy. Those surveyed discussed their reasons for taking vitamins, sometimes
claiming very specific health benefits. For one, a "high B potency"
relieved her bursitis, though she was not sure why. Another admitted that she (a registered nurse) and her husband (a physician) were sometimes "careless about balanced diets, so we
believe in the use of vitamins as supplements." Others commented that "even proper food could be vitamin deficient." However, often comments were less specific. The use of vitamins for
"health insurance" appeared frequently. Some praised the psychological effects of supplements. "When I discontinue vitamins
for my children they are cross and feel bad," explained one
mother.

These vitamin beliefs were again evident a few years later in a
survey developed to test the acceptability of specific marketing
themes for Miles Laboratories.[37] This study identified the most
acceptable physiological and psychological reasons for vitamin usage among 225 middle-income housewives, a prime market for
Miles products. From a physiological standpoint, these women accepted vitamins as a dietary supplement because they believed

that the body cannot store some vitamins, that food lacks vitamins, and that in the winter sunshine is insufficient for good health. From a psychological point of view, vitamins helped in two ways. First, they relieved homemakers' anxieties; these women were concerned about their families' well-being because they could not control what family members ate when away from home. Second, vitamin pills satisfied the homemaker's need for increased pep and energy. Throughout the 1950s and 1960s, surveys documented that both negative and positive factors impelled people to buy vitamin pills. From a negative perspective, people worried about the healthfulness of their diets; from the positive, people expected increased vitality.

In the last twenty-five years, research conducted by federal agencies such as the FDA, industry groups such as the Vitamin Nutrition Information Service of the Hoffmann-La Roche Company, and trade organizations such as the Council for Responsible Nutrition have provided more broad-based statistical studies that indicate continuity of beliefs and practices.[38] *A Study of Health Practices and Opinions*, for example, designed for the FDA, surveyed over thirty-five million adults in the early 1970s. According to the surveyors, "A large majority of the American people hold at least some inflated ideas of the benefits of taking supplemental vitamins and minerals. The most common misconception is that extra vitamins will provide more pep and energy." Despite the FDA's claims to the contrary, nearly three-fourths of the sample agreed that feeling tired and run down probably indicated the need for additional micronutrients. Seventy-eight percent believed that one should use vitamins "to stay generally more healthy."[39] The research had been designed to examine the health practices and opinions of Americans, "with particular emphasis on susceptibility to health fallacies and misrepresentations." It showed that consumers were aware of scientific controversy. In a telling description of those surveyed, the study concluded that vitamin users "showed a tendency to rely on their own judgment over conflicting opinions from physicians."[40] This depiction of vitamin users can be interpreted to mean that consumers faced with contradictory advice from physicians and researchers made up their own minds and, most significantly, that their decisions did not necessarily agree with the FDA's.

In terms of numbers, studies have estimated that 42 percent of the adult population in 1980 took vitamins regularly, between 38 percent and 41 percent in 1986, 35 percent in 1990, and 43 percent in 1993. The differences in the percentages over the years are partly a function of different survey methodologies and are less significant than the consistent demographic picture drawn of the vitamin-taking population. All the studies agreed: women were more likely to be vitamin users than men; college graduates were more likely to be vitamin users than high school graduates, who were more likely to be users than those who had not finished high school; professional, clerical, and sales people were more likely to be users than manual workers; and households at higher income levels were more likely to use vitamins as well. Moreover, those who supplemented their diets with vitamins tended to be more health-oriented in other aspects of their lives; they were less likely to smoke, exercised more, and dieted more than non-users. They were what one marketing periodical called the "take-charge" consumers, people who took responsibility for their own health.

One consequence of this attitude, applauded by *Marketing Communication,* was that "taking care" translated into supplementing the diet with vitamins.[41] Vitamins users tended to be people interested in fitness and health and concerned about diet. They were self-reliant people inclined to treat minor ailments such as sore throats and colds by themselves. It is important to emphasize that they were not anti-physician or anti-science, but they did trust their own bodies. In survey after survey and article after article, the same conclusion appeared: "Supplement usage remains a widespread behavior linked to popular conceptions of good health and well-being," and users took vitamins "to supplement their diets and for general reasons of maintaining or promoting good health."[42] Whether a national survey using a sample of thirty-five million, such as *A Study of Health Practices and Opinions,* or a small focused study using a sample of sixty patients in a single locale,[43] the results were similar. People learned about vitamin supplementation from friends, family, and nonmedical publications more often than from health-care practitioners. People believed that supplements were effective in increasing vitality and were an important form of "nutritional insurance."

Surveys give us aggregate data: 45 percent take vitamins to stay healthy, 41 percent to supplement their diet, 38 percent when exposed to colds. Missing are the voices of vitamin users, the voices we hear only rarely, for instance in letters to the FDA and the Consumers Union, voices of concerned individuals who felt that their needs were not being met. Other voices appeared at times in articles about vitamin supplementation. For example, researchers and physicians used their experiences to teach people what they believed was important about supplementation.[44] Since the topic of health is a popular subject of conversation, discussions with friends and relatives often bring out other instances.

This chorus substantiates the numerical findings of more anonymous surveys. People sometimes celebrate the successful treatment of specific conditions with vitamin supplementation, but more generally they believe that vitamins are necessary for the maintenance of their well-being and the attainment of optimal health. Though some users were alerted to the benefits of vitamins by physicians, many more learned about the micronutrients from friends, family, and the media, including advertising. One story I was told involved two sisters, one of whom took vitamins on the recommendation of a physician. A serendipitous side effect she noticed was that her horrible hangnails disappeared. On her advice, the second sister also began to use vitamin supplements; she too felt better and was no longer plagued with hangnails. If she forgot to take her daily supplement, however, they would reappear. Both readily admit that there is no likely connection between the pills and the hangnails and neither has ever read about any correlation between the two, but each is content to continue her daily routine. In another instance, a woman began taking vitamin pills when she was pregnant. She felt so good during her pregnancy that she continues the daily regimen to this day. These individual cases bring to life survey findings that the overwhelming majority of vitamin users are convinced from their own experiences that supplementation makes sense for them, that they use supplements to insure health. These and so many others who use supplements accept that we need detailed scientific studies to determine more precisely the role of vitamins in a healthy diet. But given their own experiences, they will continue to take vitamins daily, while waiting for the data.

We are all waiting for science to provide unambiguous answers to the vitamin controversy. But, as is clear from the study of vitamins in American culture, science is not a single, unalloyed body of knowledge. Interpretations of science can radically differ within a field as contentious as vitamins, as well as outside the field. Researchers used the science of vitamins to build successful research careers. Health-care professionals used the science of vitamins to enhance their professional and financial positions. Advertisers used the science of vitamins to entice consumers, especially women, to buy vitamin products. Manufacturers used the science of vitamins to build a lucrative industry. Government officials used the science of vitamins to regulate the industry. Consumers used the science of vitamins to claim control over their own health care.

As a result, despite all the research and all the analysis, we are still left with the question: "Can extra vitamins really do you any good if you eat a normal American diet?" In 1955, the answer was, "Scientists still know too little about the mysterious role that vitamins play in countless bodily processes to answer flatly yes or no, but the swing is certainly toward the affirmative."[45] Then, it seemed, science would soon disclose the answers; the vitamin industry and advertising played on this hope. Today, the answer is, we don't know "and the idea that clinical trials will give definitive answers is really holding out false hope. . . . Generations can pass before the answers are complete." Do we wait until then, or do we evaluate the totality of evidence and act on the evident trend in research results?[46] Many consumers and increasing numbers of scientists and physicians have decided not to wait and see; they are buying vitamin pills and urging others to do so as well.

For millions of American concerned about health, diet, and vitamin pills, the issues have not changed much in the past eighty years. The same claims for vitamin products, ranging from calm and measured to wild and extravagant, still appear in the press and in advertisements. The same motives, ranging from profit to protection, are still visible in our daily lives. Despite the development of increasingly sophisticated studies, we are no closer to a definitive solution to the puzzle of vitamin supplementation.

Whose science is to be believed? What science will give us sufficient evidence to make informed decisions? In the absence of harm to consumers, how far should vitamin products be controlled? How successfully could they be controlled? As individual consumers we make very personal choices. In making our decisions we must be alert to the possibilities and limitations of scientific research and the way science can be manipulated to maximize corporate gains and professional status. Science is not above commerce or politics; it is part of both. We must not allow our bodies to be the sites of profit making or power plays.

# Notes

## INTRODUCTION

1. My analysis of the use of authority of science owes much to Paul Starr's development of the concept of the cultural authority of medicine in *The Social Transformation of American Medicine: The Rise of a Sovereign Profession and the Making of a Vast Industry* (New York: Basic Books, 1982). Though the authority of science is a less focused concept than that of medicine, it radiates through American society in much the same way. Because it has a less clearly focused venue than medicine, it can be picked up and employed by a wider range of actors, as the following analysis demonstrates. See also Rima D. Apple, *Mothers and Medicine: A Social History of Infant Feeding, 1890–1950* (Madison: University of Wisconsin Press, 1987).
2. Franklin L. Chambers, "Solving the Vitamine Mystery," *Illustrated World*, Sept. 1921, p. 101.
3. Ellwood Hendrick, "Vitamines: New Light on the Mysteries of Nutrition," *Harper's Monthly Magazine*, March 1921, pp. 495–503. The standard history of nutrition research remains Elmer V. McCollum, *A History of Nutrition: The Sequence of Ideas in Nutrition Investigations* (Boston: Houghton Mifflin, 1957). See also Alesia Maltz, "The Role of Language in the Discovery and Acceptance of Vitamins" (Ph.D. diss., University of Illinois, 1989); Kenneth J. Carpenter, *The History of Scurvy and Vitamin C* (New York: Cambridge University Press, 1986); Anthony Serafini, *Linus Pauling: A Man and His Science* (New York: Simon and Schuster, 1989), Ralph W. Moss, *Free Radical: Albert Szent-Gyorgyi and the Battle of Vitamin C* (New York: Paragon, 1987).
4. Clarence Woodbury, "The A B C of Pep," *American Magazine*, Dec. 1940, pp. 23, 156–157.
5. "How One May Feast and Starve," *Literary Digest*, 19 Dec. 1914, p. 1220.
6. Myron M. Streans, "Three Times a Day," *National Weekly*, 9 May 1925, pp. 11,

45. See also Chambers, "Solving the Vitamine Mystery," p. 144; Hendrick, "Vitamines: New Light," p. 503; Woodbury, "A B C of Pep," p. 57.

7. Pellagra is another vitamin-deficiency disease that occurred in the United States in this time period. Though it was recognized as a deficiency disease, it was not listed as a vitamin-deficiency disease until 1937 when the "pellagra-preventive" was identified as nicotinic acid, or niacin. For more on this history of pellagra, see Daphne A. Roe, *A Plague of Corn: The Social History of Pellagra* (Ithaca, N.Y.: Cornell University Press, 1973).

8. Ruth F. Wadsworth, "Vitamins' Place in the Home," *Collier's*, 15 Aug. 1931, pp. 24, 27.

9. For the history of beriberi and the work that identified the necessary micronutrient, see Judith P. Swazey and Karen Reeds, "Beriberi and the Coenzyme Function of Vitamin B$_1$," in *Today's Medicine, Tomorrow's Science: Essays on Paths of Discovery in the Biomedical Sciences*, DHEW Pub. No. (NIH) 78-244 (Washington, D.C.: U.S. Department of Health, Education and Welfare, [1978]), pp. 27–51.

10. Walter H. Eddy, "Why We Need Vitamin B," *Good Housekeeping*, Nov. 1934, pp. 90, 201.

11. "Vitamins for Drinks," *Time*, 17 Jan. 1938, pp. 39–40.

12. V. V. Vitawater advertisement, *Esquire*, May 1940, p. 18.

13. "How to Keep Vitamins," *Literary Digest*, 25 March 1922, p. 25; "How to Save Vitamins," *Time*, 4 Aug. 1941, p. 48; "Vegetables as Life Insurance," *Literary Digest*, 5 April 1924, pp. 75–77; L. Jean Bogert, "Our Daily Half Dozen," *Delineator*, Feb. 1935, pp. 40–41; Eddy, "Why We Need Vitamin B," pp. 90, 201; Margaret House Irwin, "He Said She Wasn't 'On Her Toes,'" *Better Homes and Gardens*, Jan. 1934, pp. 13, 36–37; L. Jean Bogert, "Vitamins in Review," *Delineator*, Jan. 1935, pp. 26, 35.

14. Advertisement for Vitroetts, *Davenport Times*, 17 Jan. 1939, clipping located in the American Medical Association Fraud Collection, "Vitamines—Box File 279."

15. Some late twentieth-century historians have reanalyzed the data from the 1930s and concluded that the American populace was not as poorly fed as these studies purport. See, for example, Harvey Levenstein, *Paradox of Plenty: A Social History of Eating in Modern America* (New York: Oxford University Press, 1993), esp. chap. 4, pp. 53–63. However, for purposes of this study, it is not important what we think about the situation in the 1930s, but what the American populace believed. It is their conviction, or lack thereof, that might convince people they needed vitamin supplementation.

16. "Vitamin Famine Prevalent in the United States," *Science News Letter*, 22 June 1940, p. 395; W. H. Sebrell, "Nutritional Diseases in the United States," *JAMA*, 7 Sept. 1940, pp. 851–854.

17. Sebrell, "Nutritional Diseases," pp. 851–854.

18. L. Stambovsky, "The Need for Vitamins," *Consumers' Research Bulletin*, April 1942, p. 17. See also Dan Rennick, "The Potential: $496,881,000," *Drug Topics*, 5 April 1943, pp. 47, 50.

19. See chap. 2.

20. U.S. Department of Agriculture, Bureau of Human Nutrition and Home Economics, "Foods: Enriched, Restored, Fortified," Dec. 1945, slightly revised July 1946, U.S. Government Printing Office, 1946; "Vitamins: They Are Added to White Bread to Correct Dangerous Deficiencies in Nation's Diet," *Life*, 21 April 1941, pp. 65–67. See also "Vitamins at $1 a Year," *Popular Science Monthly*, Feb. 1941, p. 107, and Suzanne Rebecca White, "Chemistry and Controversy: Regulating the Use of Chemicals in Foods, 1883–1959" (Ph.D. diss., Emory University, 1994).

21. J. F. McClendon, "The Use of Vitamine Food-Tablets as an Aid Toward Conserving the Food Supply," *Science*, 28 Oct. 1921, p. 409.

22. Graham Lusk, "The Commercial Cult of Vitamins," *Survey*, 15 March 1923, pp. 784–785.

23. The *JAMA* editorial "Vitamin Theories" was reprinted in part with discussion in "What Do We Know about Vitamins?" *Literary Digest*, 26 Aug. 1922, p. 22.

24. *JAMA* editorial partially reprinted and discussed in "The Vitamins and the Jokers," *Literary Digest*, 4 July 1931, p. 19; E. J. Kohman, "Debunking the Vitamins," *Hygeia*, June 1932, 523–527.

    Medical practitioners writing about vitamin supplements typically differentiated between preparations taken under the direction of a physician and those advertised directly to the consumer. They accepted vitamins as important therapeutic items, prescribed by a physician to treat a recognized vitamin-deficiency condition. They rejected vitamin preparations that ignored physician involvement. The writings discussed in this chapter do not concern physician-prescribed vitamin supplements.

25. Sybil L. Smith, "The Vitamin Primer," *Ladies' Home Journal*, Feb. 1931, pp. 99, 113.

26. Walter H. Eddy, "Now You Can Feed Your Skin," *Good Housekeeping*, June 1938, p. 80.

27. "Vitamin Follies," *Hygeia*, February 1938, pp. 115, 172. The Federal Trade Commission evidently shared this opinion. In May 1938 it issued a complaint against the soap manufacturer; in September 1941, it ordered the company to cease and desist its claims of "beneficial value upon the skin by reason of [the soap's] vitamin content." Information about this incident can be found in the American Medical Association Fraud Collection.

28. The chronology of vitamin research can be found in McCollum, *History of Nutrition*. See also Eva D. Wilson et al., *Principles of Nutrition*, 3rd ed. (New York: John Wiley and Sons, 1975). For a contemporary analysis of the state of the field, see Randolph T. Major, "Industrial Development of Synthetic Vitamins," *Annual Report of the Smithsonian Institution*, 1942, pp. 273–288; and "Vitamin Bandwagon," *Time*, 26 April 1943, p. 36.

29. "Vitamins Reduce Lost Time in Industry," *Scientific American*, Dec. 1932, 360–361.

30. "Machine Maker Gives Vitamins to Workers," *Drug Topics*, 20 Jan. 1941, p. 12; Kenneth M. Swezey, "Industry Goes in for Vitamins to Conserve Manpower

for Defense Work," *Popular Science Monthly*, May 1942, pp. 101–107; "Vitamin Pills Cut Absences at Tool Plant," *Drug Topics*, 23 June 1941, p. 14.

31. "Industry Drafts the Vitamins," *Fortune*, Nov. 1942, pp. 64, 72; "Vitamins & Vigor," *Time*, 21 May 1945, pp. 88, 90; "Vitamin Feeding Pays," *Business Week*, 20 Feb. 1943, p. 42; "Vitamins for Workers," *Science News Letter*, 31 July 1943, pp. 76–77; "Vitamins at Work," *Newsweek*, 16 March 1943, pp. 53–54; "Vitamin Pills for Municipal Employees," *American City*, Sept. 1943, p. 15; "Pills in the Contract," *Business Week*, 16 May 1942, pp. 52–53; "Vitamin Pills Make Workers More Nutrition Conscious," *Science News Letter*, 28 Aug. 1943, p. 136.

32. Rennick, "The Potential: $496,881,000," pp. 47, 50.

33. Waldemar Kaempffert, "What We Know about Vitamins," *New York Times Magazine*, 3 May 1942, pp. 10–11, 23; Russell M. Wilder, "Hitler's Secret Weapon Is Depriving People of Vitamins," *Science News Letter*, 12 April 1941, pp. 231, 237.

34. Advertisement for Victory, *Drug Topics*, 2 March 1942, p. 17; advertisement for Vimms, *Drug Topics*, 5 April 1943, p. 51.

35. Iago Galdston, "Take Vitamins the Natural Way," *American Mercury*, Feb. 1942, pp. 223–229. See also Ruth deForest Lamb, *American Chamber of Horrors: The Truth about Food and Drugs* (New York: Farrar and Rinehart, 1936), esp. pp. 171–173; "Vitamin Merry-Go-Round," *Newsweek*, 8 Nov. 1943, p. 94.

36. Rennick, "The Potential: $496,881,000," pp. 47, 50. See also "Vitamins Go to War," *Business Week* Report to Executives, 10 July 1943, pp. 55–69.

37. For a different view of science in popular culture, one that considers the retreat of scientists from the public domain, see John C. Burnham, *How Superstition Won and Science Lost: Popularizing Science and Health in the United States* (New Brunswick, N.J.: Rutgers University Press, 1987).

## 1 POPULAR SCIENCE AND ADVERTISING

1. "The X in Food," *Independent*, 9 July 1921, p. 16. See also "The Elusive Vitamin," *Survey* 47 (1921): 368.

2. Rachel Lynn Palmer and Isidore M. Alpher, *40,000,000 Guinea Pig Children* (New York: Vanguard Press, 1937), p. 152. Similar sentiments were expressed in (Mrs.) Christine M. Frederick, *Selling Mrs. Consumer* (New York: Business Bourse, 1929); "Dr. Wiley's Question Box," *Good Housekeeping*, March 1928, p. 103. On the relationship between the science of nutrition and educated motherhood, see Rima D. Apple, "Science Gendered: Nutrition in the United States, 1840–1940," in Harmke Kamminga and Andrew Cunningham, eds., *The Science and Culture of Nutrition* (Amsterdam: Rodopi for the Wellcome Institute Series in the History of Medicine, 1995), pp. 129–154.

3. See, for example, "Vitamins," *Tide* 11, 19 (1937): 20–25, on the various ways manufacturers introduced vitamins into products.

4. Ovaltine advertisement, *Hygeia*, Dec. 1927, p. 15.

5. Kitchen Craft Waterless Cooker advertisement, *Hygeia*, Dec. 1926, p. 7.

6. Vitavose advertisement, *Good Housekeeping*, Jan. 1932, p. 102.

7. Bond Bread advertisement, *Good Housekeeping*, Feb. 1932, p. 104.

8. Vita-Ray Cream advertisement, *Good Housekeeping*, Feb. 1935, p. 232.

9. Red Heart's 3-flavor Dog Biscuits advertisement, *Parents' Magazine*, Dec. 1938, p. 96.

10. Ruth A. Guy, "The History of Cod Liver Oil as a Remedy," *American Journal of Diseases of Children* 26 (1923): 112–116; Elmer V. McCollum, *A History of Nutrition: The Sequence of Ideas in Nutrition Investigations* (Boston: Houghton Mifflin, 1957), pp. 135–137, 217–234, 271–287.

11. Alfred F. Hess, *Rickets Including Osteomalacia and Tetany* (Philadelphia: Lea and Febiger, 1929), pp. vii–viii, 17–19, 40–44. See also J. Lawson Dick, "Geographical Distribution of Rickets: Distribution in America," in *Rickets* (New York: E. B. Treat Co., 1922), pp. 56–70; Helen C. Goodspeed and Emma Johnson, *Care and Training of Children* (Philadelphia: J. B. Lippincott, 1929), p. 82; and *Holt's Diseases of Infancy and Childhood: A Textbook for the Use of Students and Practitioners*, 10th ed., rev. by L. Emmett Holt, Jr., and Rustin McIntosh (New York: D. Appleton-Century, 1936).

12. Marguerite Gauger, "Sunlight Rain or Shine," *Parents' Magazine*, Jan. 1933, pp. 26, 35; Nicholas and Lillian Kopeloff, "Vitamin Preparation or Victuals?" *New Republic*, 23 Aug. 1922, pp. 353–355; Martha Elliot, "Sunlight for Babies," *Child Health Bulletin* 1 (1925): 35–38; Josephine Hemenway Kenyon, "New Ideas for Scientific Motherhood," *Good Housekeeping*, Sept. 1925, p. 92; and Jerome E. Ephriam, "The Truth about Vitamins," *American Mercury* 36 (1935): 490–492.

13. Palmer and Alpher, *40,000,000 Guinea Pig Children*, p. 8.

14. Russell M. Wilder, "Food Facts and Fallacies," *Hygeia*, July 1938, p. 629.

15. "Slogan," *Tide* 9, 1 (1935): 71.

16. "Among Hygeia Advertisers," *Hygeia*, Dec. 1926, p. 2.

17. Walter H. Eddy, "At Your Service: The Story of the Good Housekeeping Bureau," *Good Housekeeping*, May 1935, pp. 92, 268–270.

18. Darrell B. Lucas and C. E. Benson, "Historical Trends of Negative-Appeals in Advertising," *Journal of Applied Psychology*, Aug. 1929, pp. 346–356; Carl A. Naether, *Advertising to Women* (New York: Prentice-Hall, 1928), pp. 153–154; Stephen Fox, *The Mirror Makers: A History of American Advertising and Its Creators* (New York: Vintage Books, 1984); T. J. Jackson Lears, "From Salvation to Self-Realization: Advertising and the Therapeutic Roots of the Consumer Culture, 1880–1930," in Richard Wightman Fox and T. J. Jackson Lears, eds., *The Culture of Consumption: Critical Essays in American History, 1880–1980* (New York: Pantheon, 1983), pp. 1–38.

19. Effective promotional campaigns present situations recognizable to the consumer. Not that advertisements are, or should strive to be, replicates of the world around us. Rather, they are reflections of reality, or more accurately reflections of desired reality. To quote one historian of advertising, "To stay effective, advertising could not depart too far from established public tastes and habits: consumers might be nudged but still balk at being shoved. Ads

necessarily *reflected* the times, and as an independent force they helped *shape* the times. . . . Advertising thus was always both mirror and mindbender" (Fox, *The Mirror Makers*, p. 64).

20. Rima D. Apple, "Constructing Mothers: Scientific Motherhood in the Nineteenth and Twentieth Centuries," *Social History of Medicine* 8 (1995): 161–178.

21. Clearly advertising did not create and impose on consumers the ideology of scientific motherhood. However, the mass of advertising using this ideology, both tacitly and overtly, served to reinforce and reproduce scientific motherhood in the culture. For more on this point, see Rima D. Apple, *Mothers and Medicine: A Social History of Infant Feeding, 1890–1950* (Madison: University of Wisconsin Press, 1987), esp. chaps. 6–9; and idem, "Constructing Mothers."

22. Samuel J. Thomas, "Nostrum Advertising and the Image of Woman as Invalid in Late Victorian America," *Journal of American Culture*, 5, 3 (1982): 104–112; Rima D. Apple, "Advertised by Our Loving Friends: The Infant Formula Industry and the Creation of New Pharmaceutical Markets, 1870–1910," *Journal of the History of Medicine*, Jan. 1986, pp. 3–23.

23. Cream of Wheat advertisement, *Parents' Magazine*, Feb. 1934, p. 31; "Fortify Your Children," *Tide* 6, 2 (1932): 22.

24. Squibb's Cod-Liver Oil advertisement, *Good Housekeeping*, Feb. 1926, p. 145.

25. Squibb's Cod-Liver Oil advertisement, *Good Housekeeping*, Dec. 1926, p. 249.

26. Oscodal advertisement, *Hygeia*, Dec. 1928, p. 13. Funk created Oscodal for the Metz Company. The product was the first concentrated vitamin approved by the AMA. Benjamin Harrow, *Casimir Funk: Pioneer in Vitamins and Hormones* (New York: Dodd, Mead, 1955), pp. 56–64, 131–132.

27. McKesson's Cod Liver Oil advertisement, *Good Housekeeping*, Mar. 1936, p. 243.

28. "Among Hygeia Advertisers," *Hygeia*, Dec. 1928, p. 2.

29. McKesson's Cod Liver Oil advertisement, *Good Housekeeping*, Mar. 1936, p. 243.

30. "Jag Over," *Tide* 6, 12 (1932): 11–12; Canned pineapple advertisement, *Hygeia*, Feb. 1933, p. 179.

31. "Boost for Bread," *Tide* 8, 4 (1934): 54.

32. Nason's Cod Liver Oil advertisement, *Hygeia*, Oct. 1928, p. 33.

33. Squibb's Cod-Liver Oil advertisement, *Good Housekeeping*, March 1939, p. 108.

34. Abbott's Cod Liver Oil advertisement, *Hygeia*, Dec. 1930, p. 1081.

35. Lysol advertisement, *Good Housekeeping*, May 1936, p. 107.

36. Squibb's Cod-Liver Oil advertisement, *Parents' Magazine*, Nov. 1936, p. 2.

37. White's Cod Liver Oil advertisement, *Hygeia*, Dec. 1930, p. 1095.

38. Squibb Adex Tablets-10 D advertisement, *Good Housekeeping*, Nov. 1932, p. 105.

39. McKesson's Cod Liver Oil advertisement, *Good Housekeeping*, Oct. 1934, p. 17740.

40. McKesson's Cod Liver Oil advertisement, *Parents' Magazine*, Nov. 1935, p. 53.

41. "Vitamins," *Tide* 11, 19 (1937): 20.

42. Interestingly, Vitamins Plus's place of sale points to another issue that warrants further research. Pharmacists for decades had been coping with attempts by the medical profession to define and limit the pharmacist's role. With products such as Vitamins Plus selling in grocery and department stores, pharmacists feared further encroachment, this time on the commercial side. In some states pharmacy boards sued to prohibit the sale of vitamins outside of drugstores. See chap. 3.

43. Vitamins Plus advertisement, *Drug Topics*, 22 Jan. 1940, p. 9.

44. Advertisements for Vitamins Plus can be found in contemporary newspapers and women's magazine such as *Harper's Bazaar* and *Good Housekeeping*. Clippings of many of these are now located in the "Vitamins Plus" file of the Food and Drug Administration Archives, RG88 Acc. no. 63A292, box 480.

45. "Beauty building from A to G," circular sent to the Food and Drug Administration by W.R.H., 15 Jan. 1938, located in the "Vitamins Plus" file of the Food and Drug Administration Archives, RG88 Acc. no. 63A292, box 480.

46. Letter from W.R.H., 8 Jan. 1938, and reply from J. J. Durrett, M.D., chief of the Drug Division, FDA, both located in the "Vitamins Plus" file of the Food and Drug Administration Archives, RG88 Acc. no. 63A292, box 480. Other letters from concerned consumers and pharmacy leaders as well can be found in this file.

47. Memo from FDA Drug Division to Chief, Eastern Division, 19 Aug. 1938, located in the "Vitamins Plus" file of the Food and Drug Administration Archives, RG88 Acc. no. 63A292, box 480.

48. Memo from P. B. Dunbar to the Federal Trade Commission, 11 Jan. 1939, in response to letter from W. F. Davidson, acting director of the Radio and Periodical Division, Federal Trade Commission, 10 Dec. 1938, located in the "Vitamins Plus" file of the Food and Drug Administration Archives, RG88 Acc. no. 63A292, box 480.

49. "Trade Commission Cases," *New York Times*, 24 Oct. 1940. A copy of the Stipulation (02652) is also located in the "Vitamins Plus" file of the Food and Drug Administration Archives, RG88 Acc. no. 63A292, box 480.

50. "Vitamin Vistas," *Tide* 12, 13 (1938): 22–23; "Vitamins," *Tide* 12, 18 (1938): 9–11; "Again, Vitamins," *Tide* 12, 23 (1938): 11–12.

51. R.E.D., in a letter dated 4 Feb. 1960, complained to the FDA that her name had been put on a Vitamins Plus mailing list. Her letter and the FDA's reply are located in the "Vitamins Plus" file of the Food and Drug Administration Archives, RG88 Acc. no. 63A292, box 480.

52. Herman Kogan, *The Long White Line: The Story of Abbott Laboratories* (New York: Random House, 1963), pp. 144, 148; Samuel Mines, *Pfizer: An Informal History* (New York: Pfizer, 1978), pp. 51–61, 66; Leonard Engel, *Medicine Makers of Kalamazoo* (New York: McGraw-Hill, 1961), pp. 77–79.

53. "Vitamins Go to War," *Business Week*, 10 July 1943, pp. 56–69.

54. "Vitamins," *Tide* 12, 18 (1938): 10; "Again, Vitamins," *Tide* 12, 23 (1938): 11. "Vitamins, vitamins," *New Republic*, 11 Jan. 1939, p. 272. Additional statistics may be found in "Vitamins Get a Book of Rules," *Business Week*, 6 April 1940,

pp. 40–43; "The Vitamin Industry," *Scientific American*, April 1941, p. 209; T. Swann Harding, "What about Vitamin Tablets," *Scientific American*, May 1943, p. 214; and "The Vitamin Business," *Fortune*, May 1945, pp. 140–142, 166, 168, 170, 172, 175.

55. The scope and content of today's market can be gauged from current editions of *Physicians' Desk Reference for Nonprescription Drugs* (Oradell, N.J.: Medical Economics Co.).

56. "Supplements Aren't Superior," *Wisconsin State Journal*, 26 Jan. 1986, sec. 5, p. 4; "The Vitamin Pushers," *Consumer Reports*, March 1986, p. 170; Council for Responsible Nutrition, "Dietary Supplement Retail Sales, 1976–1993," *1993 Overview of the Nutritional Supplement Market* (Washington, D.C.: CRN, 1994); Miriam Shuchman and Michael Wilkes, "The Vitamin Uprising," *New York*, 2 Oct. 1994, p. 79.

57. Bonnie Liebman, "Vitamin Supplements," *Nutrition Action*, Feb. 1986, p. 5. For more on contemporary advertising techniques and theory, see Raymond Williams, "Advertising: The Magic System," in *Problems in Materialism and Culture* (New York: Schocken, 1980) pp. 170–195; and Judith Williamson, *Decoding Advertisements: Ideology and Meaning in Advertising* (New York: Marion Boyars, 1978).

## 2 VITAMINS, MARKETING, AND RESEARCH

1. Robert Taylor, "The Birth of the Wisconsin Alumni Research Foundation," typescript dated 1956, in the files of the Wisconsin Alumni Research Foundation, hereafter referred to as WARF files.

2. H. Steenbock and A. Black, "Fat-Soluble Vitamins: The Induction of Growth-Promoting and Calcifying Properties in a Ration by Exposure to Ultra-Violet Light," *Journal of Biological Chemistry* 61 (1924): 405–422; H. Steenbock, "Special Articles: The Induction of Growth Promoting and Calcifying Properties in a Ration by Exposure to Light," *Science* 60 (1924): 224–225. See Letter to the Editor, *JAMA*, 19 July 1930, p. 220; and [Harry Steenbock], "Excerpts from Publications and Copies of Correspondence Relating to the Priority of the Discovery of Antirachitic Activation and the Reactions of Dr. Hess to Patent Application: A Reply to the Comments of Mr. Auerbacher on an Article by Paul DeKruif Published in the *Ladies' Home Journal*, May 1935," University of Wisconsin Archives, Harry Steenbock General Subject Files, 9/11/13/3, box 15. The Steenbock General Subject Files, 9/11/13/3, will hereafter be referred to as Steenbock General. To a large extent, conflicting priority claims resulted from different definitions of what constituted the "discovery" of ultraviolet effects. For an analogous situation in other vitamin research, see Naomi Aronson, "Resistance to Discovery: Vitamins, History, and Careers," *Isis* 77 (1986): 630–646.

3. Information about Steenbock's life has been drawn from two primary sources: Howard Schneider, "Harry Steenbock (1886–1967)—A Biographical Sketch," *Journal of Nutrition* 103 (1973): 1233–1247; and an interview

with Aaron Ihde, professor emeritus, University of Wisconsin, and former student of Steenbock, conducted 5 Feb. 1988. I thank Prof. Ihde for the time he took to discuss Steenbock's life and work with me. See also Mark H. Ingraham, *Charles Sumner Slichter: The Golden Vector* (Madison: University of Wisconsin Press, 1972), pp. 176–179.

4. For more on the relationship between "pure" and "applied" science in schools of agriculture and agricultural experiment stations at this time, see Charles E. Rosenberg, "Science Pure and Science Applied: Two Studies in the Social Origin of Scientific Research," pp. 185–195 in his *No Other Gods: On Science and American Social Thought* (Baltimore: Johns Hopkins University Press, 1976).

5. Harry Steenbock, "The Relations of the Writer to the Wisconsin Alumni Research Foundation," Jan. 1926, p. 4, University of Wisconsin Archives, Harry Steenbock WARF Special Files, 9/11/13/1, box 1. The Steenbock WARF Special Files, 9/11/13/1, files will hereafter be referred to as Steenbock WARF. For more on the patenting of insulin, see Michael Bliss, *The Discovery of Insulin* (Chicago: University of Chicago Press, 1982), esp. pp. 131–133, 137–139, 174–181.

6. Steenbock, "Relations."

7. Ihde, interview; Schneider, "Harry Steenbock"; Steenbock, "Relations," p. 5.

8. F. B. Morrison to H. L. Russell, 14 Dec. 1925, WARF files.

9. A. J. Glover to Russell, 22 Oct. 1925, WARF files; Morrison to Russell, 14 Dec. 1925, WARF files.

10. F. B. Morrison to Russell, 28 Oct. 1925, WARF files; Edward H. Beardsley, *Harry L. Russell and Agricultural Science in Wisconsin* (Madison: University of Wisconsin Press, 1969), p. 160; and Ihde, interview.

11. Morrison to Russell, 28 Oct. 1925, WARF files.

12. For more on the role of scientists at public institutions and the tension between the push of research and the pull of social and commercial considerations, see Rosenberg, *No Other Gods*, particularly part 2; and Charles Weiner, "Universities, Professors and Patents: A Continuing Controversy," *Technology Review* (Feb.-Mar. 1986): 33–43.

13. H. L. Russell, "The Wisconsin Alumni Research Foundation: Its Purpose," typescript dated Feb. 1931, WARF files; Beardsley, *Harry L. Russell*, p. 157.

14. F. B. Morrison to Russell, 28 Oct. 1925, WARF files.

15. M. K. Hobbs to Steenbock, 9 Feb. 1929, Steenbock WARF, box 1.

16. H. E. Gunn to Steenbock, 24 April 1929, Steenbock WARF, box 1.

17. "Eating and Drinking Sunshine!" found in Steenbock General, box 15.

18. Joseph P. Sereda, trading under the name and style of Health Violet Products, Docket 1695, *Federal Trade Commission Decisions*, vol. 13, pp. 134–140.

19. "Vitamin Ads under Fire," *Business Week*, 27 Dec. 1937, pp. 49–50.

20. Russell, "Wisconsin Alumni Research Foundation," p. 22.

21. Steenbock antirachitic product and process (basic) 1,680,818, 14 Aug. 1928; antirachitic product and process (cereals) 1,871,135, 9 Aug. 1932; antirachitic

product and process (essence) 1,871,136, 9 Aug. 1932 and antirachitic product and process (yeast) 2,057,399, 13 Oct. 1936.

22. Steenbock, "Relations," p. 3.

23. Harry Steenbock, "The Administration of the Results of Research," undated typescript, pp. 6–7, Steenbock WARF, box 1.

24. Steenbock to Russell, 17 Dec. 1925, WARF files; Marvin to Steenbock, 17 March 1923, Steenbock WARF, box 2.

25. At this time, other universities were becoming involved in patenting arrangements. The Regents of the University of California created a patent-management corporation. At the University of Minnesota, the Board of Regents processed its patents. Columbia University established University Patents, Inc., which entered into agreements with a nonprofit foundation Research Corporation. For more on university research patenting in the period, see Rima D. Apple, "Patenting University Research: Harry Steenbock and the Wisconsin Alumni Research Foundation," *Isis* 80 (1989): 375–394; Archie M. Palmer, *Survey of University Patent Policies: Preliminary Report* (Washington, D.C.: National Research Council, 1948); Archie M. Palmer, *University Patent Policies and Practices* (Washington, D.C.: National Research Council of the National Academy of Sciences, 1952); Beardsley, *Harry L. Russell*, pp. 155–158; Steenbock, "Relations," pp. 3–4; Schneider, "Harry Steenbock," p. 1244; Ingraham, *Charles Sumner Slichter*, pp. 178–179. See also William Alan Richardson, "Research: Self-Supporting," *Medical Economics*, Dec. 1935, pp. 15–18.

26. Steenbock to Haight, 7 Dec. 1929, University of Wisconsin Archives, E. B. Fred Files, 4/16/4, box 50 (hereafter referred to as the Fred Files).

27. Beardsley, *Harry L. Russell*, pp. 157–158, citing university business manager James Phillips, quoted in *Madison* (Wisc.) *Capital Times*, 8 March 1938.

28. For more on Steenbock's experiences with the Board of Regents and the vitamin A patent, see Steenbock, "Relations"; Steenbock to C. A. Dykstra, 1 Dec. 1942, Steenbock WARF, box 2; E. B. Fred, "The Years of Decision: The Early Years of the Wisconsin Alumni Research Foundation," typescript history dated March 1960, archive copy in University of Wisconsin Archives; A. B. Marvin to Steenbock, 17 March 1923, Steenbock WARF, box 2; Steenbock to Russell, 17 Dec. 1925, WARF files.

29. Steenbock to WARF Trustees, 13 June 1928, Steenbock WARF, box 2; memorandum concerning federal appropriations supporting agricultural research at the University of Wisconsin, typescript dated 30 Oct. 1933, Steenbock WARF, box 2; "WARF Report," reprinted from *The Wisconsin Alumnus,* June 1948, in Steenbock WARF, box 2; Russell to Pres. E. A. Birge, 16 April 1925, WARF files; Steenbock to Haight, 7 Dec. 1929, WARF files; Richardson, "Research: Self-Supporting," pp. 15–18; Beardsley, *Harry L. Russell.*

Russell, one of WARF's most ardent supporters, explained how he saw the foundation managing patents for the public good:

1. protecting discoveries from crass commercialism;

2. using licensure to control the quality of the products and their advertising;
3. granting limited licensing to minimize the monopolistic character of patents;
4. applying profits to further university research.

"In a word," he wrote in 1931, "we are hoping to retain all of the social advantages that may come to the public and at the same time handle the business to be developed with something of the efficiency which at least theoretically obtains from private corporate control. We recognize the experimental nature of this effort to socialize these values." Russell, "The Wisconsin Alumni Research Foundation."

30. [Slichter] to W. S. Kies, 6 Oct. 1925, Steenbock WARF, box 2.
31. For correspondence about the Quaker Oats contract, see Steenbock, WARF, box 1; Fred, "Years of Decision"; Taylor, "Birth of the Wisconsin Alumni Research Foundation."
32. For a discussion of the uses of cod-liver oil, see chap. 1.
33. G.H.A. Clowes, Director of Research, Lilly Research Laboratories, to H. B. Steenbock, 29 Oct. 1924, Steenbock WARF, box 1; Steenbock to E. H. Volwiler, Abbott Laboratories, 6 Jan. 1925, University of Wisconsin Archives, Harry Steenbock General Correspondence Files, 9/11/13/2, box 1-A (hereafter referred to as Steenbock Correspondence); Clowes to Steenbock, 6 March 1925, Steenbock WARF, box 1; Haight to Steenbock, 27 March 1928, Steenbock WARF, box 1; Steenbock to W. S. Kies, 28 June 1928, Steenbock WARF, box 1; Steenbock to Haight, 10 Oct. 1928, Steenbock WARF, box 1; Steenbock to L. M. Hanks, 10 Oct. 1928, Steenbock WARF, box 1; M. K. Hobbs to Steenbock, 22 Oct. 1928, Steenbock WARF, box 1; Parke, Davis & Co. to Haight, 29 Dec. 1928, Steenbock WARF, box 1; Steenbock to Hanks, 29 Jan. 1929, Steenbock WARF, box 1; Steenbock to Carroll Dunham Smith Pharmaceutical Co., 25 April 1929, Steenbock WARF, box 1; Steenbock to Gunn, 27 Nov. 1929, Steenbock WARF, box 1; and Gunn to Steenbock, 29 Nov. 1929, Steenbock WARF, box 1.

Other pharmaceutical companies denied use of the Steenbock process looked for alternatives. Upjohn, for example, attempted to irradiate by sunlight. The large trays of ergosterol that were set out in fields in the sunny southwest did produce vitamin D, but high costs made this method commercially unfeasible. As manufacturers were aware, the vitamin D potency of cod liver and other fish oils varies tremendously. By 1936 Upjohn had discovered that the most potent oil came from Iceland. Six months of careful assaying proved that the best oil came from cod caught off the north coast of Iceland during the autumn. At about the same time, the International Vitamin Corporation of New York had found that ethylene dichloride dissolved vitamin D and could extract vitamin D from cod-liver oil. Upjohn obtained an exclusive U.S. license for the concentrating process and employed it to produce a concentrate from the extra-potent Icelandic cod-liver oil. Using this concentrate to manufacture capsules and commercial liquid concentrates, Upjohn successfully competed in the vitamin D market, even without the Steenbock process. Leonard Engel, *Medicine Makers of Kalamazoo* (New York: McGraw-Hill, 1961), pp. 70–74; Steenbock to Edward S. Rogers, 2 Jan. 1930, Steenbock WARF, box 1; and Audrey Davis, "The Rise of the Vitamin-Medicinal as Illustrated by Vitamin D," *Pharmacy in History* 24 (1982): 59–72.

34. Steenbock to Carroll Dunham Smith Pharmaceutical Co., 25 April 1929, Steenbock WARF, box 1.

35. See, for example, Steenbock General, box 13; Steenbock General, box 16.

36. See, for example, Steenbock to Gunn, 27 Nov. 1929, Steenbock WARF, box 1; Steenbock to L. M. Hanks, 17 Sept. 1930, Steenbock WARF, box 3.

37. H. W. Hibbard to Steenbock, 14 Aug. 1929, Steenbock WARF, box 1.

38. Steenbock to C. E. Wheelock Co., Peoria, Ill., 28 Feb. 1929, Steenbock WARF, box 1.

39. F. B. Morrison to Russell, 28 Oct. 1925, and Morrison to Russell, 14 Dec. 1925, WARF files; Steenbock, "Relations."

40. Steenbock to C. A. Dykstra, 1 Dec. 1942, Steenbock WARF, box 2; Steenbock to Christensen, 30 Nov. 1942, Steenbock WARF, box 2.

41. Milk report no. 25, 31 March 1941; Milk Report no. 8, 20 April 1935; Milk report no. 9, 27 July 1935; Milk Report no. 10, 22 Oct. 1935; Milk Report no. 13, 26 June 1936; Milk Report no. 14, 15 Aug. 1936; Milk Report no. 16, 20 Jan. 1937; Milk Report no. 18, 23 Aug. 1937; Milk Report no. 22, 21 Oct. 1938; Milk Report no. 20, 21 Jan. 1938; Milk Report no. 23, 25 March 1939; all Milk Reports found in Steenbock WARF, box 2; third annual report of the Director of WARF, 1932, Steenbock WARF, box 2; Evan A. Evans to Trustees, 26 March 1934, Steenbock WARF, box 3.

42. Milk Report no. 13, 26 June 1936, Steenbock WARF, box 2.

43. Fred, "Years of Decision," pp. 23–24, quoting the minutes of the Board of Trustees, 18 Feb. 1927 and 22 June 1929; Steenbock to Slichter, 24 March 1928, Steenbock WARF, box 2.

44. Steenbock to Mory, 6 Jan. 1923, and Mory to Steenbock, 20 Dec. 1922, Steenbock Correspondence, box 1.

45. Steenbock to Fine, 22 Sept. 1924, Steenbock WARF, box 1.

46. Steenbock to Kletzien, 6 May 1936; memo Kletzien to Steenbock, undated; Alfred E. Bott, "Brewers Are Turning to Vitamins," *Modern Brewer*, April 1936, pp. 44–46, all in Steenbock WARF, box 2.

47. Archie M. Palmer, *Nonprofit Research and Patent Management in the United States*, Pub. 371 (Washington, D.C.: National Academy of Science-National Research Council, 1956).

48. Initially an inventor would receive 15 percent of the royalties and WARF the remainder. These proportions have changed over the years. Today inventors receive 20 percent and the inventor's department 15 percent; the remainder becomes part of WARF's pool of resources.

49. For more on the financial success of WARF, see Apple, "Patenting University Research."

50. H. A. Toulmin, Jr., "Commercial Research by Universities Threatens Science

and Education," *Product Engineering*, June 1947, reprint located in Steenbock General, box 16. See also "Report of the Committee on Clinical Investigations and Scientific Research," *Journal of Pediatrics* 8 (1936): 124–130.

51. "Proposed Statement by Mr. Haight," typescript, c. 1946, Steenbock WARF, box 2; "The Steenbock Patents," *Drug Trade News*, 19 July 1943, clipping in Steenbock WARF, box 2; "Court Withdraws Ruling against Steenbock Patents," *New York Herald Tribune*, 23 Aug. 1943, clipping in the Fred Files.

52. Steenbock to H. C. Jackson, 20 July 1939, Steenbock WARF, box 1.

53. Today patenting has become the norm on campuses all across the country. While WARF serves as a model of successful university-associated patent-management, it is not obvious that WARF's prosperity can be duplicated today. For more on these points, see Apple, "Patenting University Research"; Dorothy Nelkin, *Science as Intellectual Property: Who Controls Research?*, AAAS Series on Issues in Science and Technology (New York: Macmillan, 1984); Martin Kenney, *Biotechnology: The University-Industrial Complex* (New Haven: Yale University Press, 1986); Irwin Feller, "University Patent and Technology-Licensing Strategies," *Educational Policy* 4 (1990): 327–340; David Blumenthal et al., "Commercializing University Research: Lessons from the Experience of the Wisconsin Alumni Research Foundation," *New England Journal of Medicine*, 19 June 1986, pp. 1621–1626.

54. In a contemporary recasting of this issue of control to protect the public, Patrick Kelly, a St. Louis attorney, engineer, and writer, has obtained a patent for a lifesupport machine to support bodyless heads. He is not building the machine but patented the plans "in order to prevent anyone from building and using such equipment without a full public debate." Carolyn Levi, "Patent Probes Ethics of Keeping Severed Head Alive," *Madison* (Wisc.) *Capital Times*, 24 Feb. 1988.

## 3 PHARMACISTS, GROCERS, PHYSICIANS, AND LINUS PAULING

1. "Vitamins and Chains," *Tide* 13, 3 (1939), pp. 38–42.

2. "Pharmacists Glean Data on Vitamins," *Drug Topics*, 10 Aug. 1936, p. 20; Jud Carrol, "Vitamins Go Multiple," *Druggists Circular*, March 1939, pp. 22–23, 82, 87; idem, "Vitamins to Go," *Druggists Circular*, March 1939, pp. 22–23, 87, 90.

3. "4,000 Grocery Outlets Sell Vitamin Capsules," *Drug Topics*, 13 March 1939, pp. 3, 34.

4. My analysis of the case is drawn from the case records, case no. 16637 of the Indiana Appellate Court. I would like to thank the Indiana Commission on Public Records, Archives Division, for sending me copies of these records. Microfilm copies of these records are available at the archives. See also "Validity of 1927 Pharmacy Law Contested by Kroger's," *Indiana Pharmacy*, April 1939, p. 129; "Vitamins," *Tide* 13, 11 (1939), p. 28.

5. Stephens Rippey, "Food Chain Wants Vitamin Sale Okay," *Drug Topics*, 28 Oct. 1940, pp. 2, 11.

6. "APhA-NARD Hit Vitamin Rule," *Drug Topics*, 11 Nov. 1940, pp. 2, 12.

7. See chaps. 6–8 for the Food and Drug Administration and vitamin regulation.

8. "Fight to Hold Vitamin Sales against Grocery Competition," *Druggists Circular*, Sept. 1939, pp. 16–17, 62.

9. "Editorial: Vitamin Promotion," *Drug Topics*, 25 May 1942, p. 16.

10. "Department of State et al *v* Kroger Grocery & Baking Company," *Reports of the Cases Decided in the Supreme Court of Indiana*, vol. 221, from 25 Jan. 1943, to 22 Nov. 1943, pp. 44–47; "Flash! Vitamin Case Ruling," *Indiana Pharmacist*, Feb. 1943, pp. 44–45; "Indiana Supreme Court Ruling Restores Board Curb on Vitamin Sales," *Drug Topics*, 8 March 1943, pp. 3, 12.

11. "Indiana Puts Vitamins into 2 General Groups," *Drug Topics*, 15 Nov. 1943, p. 3.

12. See, for the example of New Jersey, "Jersey Board to Appeal Ruling on Sale of Vitamin Capsules," *Drug Topics*, 18 Nov. 1940, pp. 3, 17; "Vitamins—Foods or Drugs?" *Consumers' Digest*, Feb. 1941, pp. 1–7. For other states, see "Vitamin Ruling Fought," *Business Week*, 23 Dec. 1944, p. 96; "Utah Limits Medical Vitamin Sale," *Drug Topics*, 10 Jan. 1944, p. 32; "Utah Orders All Medicinal Vitamins to Be Sold Only in Drug Stores," *Drug Topics*, 24 Jan. 1944, pp. 2, 6; "Utah Medicinal Vitamin Line Holds as Non-Drug Outlets Launch Attack," *Drug Topics*, 21 Feb. 1944, pp. 3, 10; "Minn. Legal Chief: Vitamin Concentrates Are Not Food," *Drug Topics*, 1 May 1944, pp. 2, 34; AGMA [Associated Grocery Manufacturers of America]—Legal Bulletin—1940: Re: Retail Sale of Vitamin Products, 18 March 1940 (copy in the FDA Archives, RG88, Acc. no. 59A2736, box 29).

13. See, in State of New York, *Annual Report of the Attorney-General for the Year Ending December 31, 1944* (Albany: William Press, 1945), pp. 226–229, a letter dated 22 June 1944, from Attorney General Nathaniel L. Goldstein, in response to query from Dr. Leslie C. Jayne, secretary of the State Board of Pharmacy. See also "Vitamin Tablets are Ruled Drugs and General Sale in State Curbed," *New York Times*, 24 June 1944; "Curbs Vitamin Sales," *Business Week*, 1 July 1944, pp. 88, 90; "Vitamins Are Not Groceries," *Newsweek*, 3 July 1944, p. 75; "N.Y. Limits Vitamin Sales to Drug Stores in State," *Drug Topics*, 10 July 1944, pp. 2, 20; "Vitamin Ruling Fought," *Business Week*, 23 Dec. 1944, p. 96.

14. "Vitamin Ruling Questioned: Attorney General's Opinion Regarded as Without Scientific Basis," *New York Times*, 24 June 1944.

15. "Editorial: Are Vitamins Drugs?" *New York Times*, 6 July 1944.

16. "Food Men Sure on N.Y. Vitamin Ruling," *Drug Topics*, 25 Dec. 1944, p. 2; "Editorial: Vitamin Court Action," *Drug Topics*, 8 Jan. 1945, p. 34.

17. "Food Retailers, Suit Upheld on Vitamin Ruling," *New York Herald Tribune*, 2 March 1945; "Vitamin Court Fight Looms as N.Y. Board Loses Plea," *Drug Topics*, 19 March 1945, p. 2.

18. "Sends Inquiries to Physicians, Increases His Vitamin Business," *Drug Topics*, 3 Feb. 1941, p. 25.

19. "Bases Vitamin Merchandising on Needs of Customer, Not on Price," *Drug Topics*, 7 Feb. 1944, p. 42.

20. "Avoidance of Indiscriminate Vitamin Selling Wins Trust," *Drug Topics*, 1 May 1944, p. 53.

21. "Newark Stores to Observe February as Vitamin Month," *Drug Topics*, 27 Jan. 1941, p. 26.

22. "'Know Your Vitamins' Drive Wins Patrons from Non-Drug Outlets," *Drug Topics*, 3 Nov. 1941, p. 31; "Chart in Window Informs Patrons on Vitamin Needs," *Drug Topics*, 3 Nov. 1941, p. 39; "N.J. Druggists to Repeat 'Vitamin Month' Drive," *Drug Topics*, 19 Feb. 1945, p. 59.

23. See, for example, Grove's advertisements in *Drug Topics*, 9 Feb. 1942, pp. 8–9.

24. *Drug Topics*, 19 April 1963, p. 30.

25. *Drug Topics*, 5 April 1943, pp. 28–29, and 29 March 1943, pp. 10–11.

26. Statistics were published each year in *Drug Topics*, usually in June and August for the previous year. Unfortunately, the figures are not always comparable or analyzed in the same categories.

27. "California Druggists Are Up in Arms on Plan to License Vitamin Dealers," *Drug Topics*, 2 April 1945, pp. 2, 38.

28. "California Board Warns Grocers against Sales of Vitamin Products," *Drug Topics*, 25 Aug. 1952, pp. 2, 55.

29. "Fight looms on grocers' move to sell drug items," *Drug Topics*, 10 Aug. 1942, p. 4; "California Board Cites Food Stores for Vitamin Sales," *Drug Topics*, 28 Sept. 1942, p. 2; "California Board Warns Grocers against Sales of Vitamin Products," *Drug Topics*, 25 Aug. 1952, pp. 2, 55; "Therapeutic Vitamins Limited to Drug Stores by California, *Drug Topics*, 15 June 1953, pp. 3, 90.

30. "Calif. Upholds Restriction on Dose Vitamins," *Drug Topics*, 22 Feb. 1954, p. 2.

31. "Recommending Vitamin Products Isn't Prescribing, Calif. Man Says," *Drug Topics*, 8 March 1954, p. 16.

32. "Editorial: Push Vitamins," *Drug Topics*, 10 June 1957, p. 44.

33. "What Customers Spent . . . ," *Drug Topics*, 17 July 1961, p. 2.

34. John A. Lynch, "You're an Expert on Vitamins," *Drug Topics*, 6 Feb. 1967, p. 4.

35. "Editorial: Vitamin Push," *Drug Topics*, 3 June 1963. See also the accompanying editorial cartoon entitled "The 'Answer Man.'"

36. "Advertising Campaign Backs Squibb 'Vigran,'" *Drug Topics*, 8 Oct. 1962; "NY Co-op Ad Program Launched by Squibb," *Drug News Weekly*, 24 July 1963, p. 4; Squibb advertisement, *Drug News Weekly*, 6 March 1963, p. 24.

37. The proportion of vitamin sales to total drugstore sales was reported periodically in *Drug Topics*.

38. "Vitamins Charge Hits at Rough Time," *Drug News Weekly*, 4 March 1964.

39. "Marketeers View '82," *Advertising Age*, 4 Jan. 1982, pp. 2, 46–48, 50–51; Martha Glaser, "Rising above the Economy," *Drug Topics*, 5 July 1972, pp. 6–10, 43, 46; Jube Shiver, Jr., "As Vitamin Sales Pep up, So Do Worries on Overuse," *Los Angeles Times*, 23 March 1986.

40. Council for Responsible Nutrition, *1993 Overview of the Nutritional Supplement Market* (Washington, D.C.: CRN, 1994), esp. "1993 Vitamin & Mineral Class of Trade" chart, p. 8.

41. Books could be written about Pauling and his relationship with the medical profession. I focus on one aspect, the controversy over vitamin C therapy and colds as portrayed in the popular media. Most Americans do not read medical literature regularly and they form their opinions and buying habits more on the popular media than the medical press. For Pauling and the medical profession from a medical orientation, see Evelleen Richards, *Vitamin C and Cancer: Medicine or Politics?* (New York: St. Martin's Press, 1991).

42. See, for example, "Vitamins—Health's Mysterious Allies," *Popular Mechanics*, Nov. 1930, pp. 722–727; Hugh Chaplin, "Vitamins: What They Are and What They Do," *Parents' Magazine*, March 1932, pp. 30, 68–69; Gulielma F. Alsop, "Fighting Winter with Food," *Woman's Journal*, Dec. 1929, pp. 46, 48.

43. "Vitamins Reduce Lost Time in Industry," *Scientific American*, Dec. 1932, pp. 360–361.

44. "Explain Function of Vitamin Items to All Prospects," *Drug Topics*, 20 Nov. 1939, p. 27; Joseph Jay Gold, "Voice of the Druggist: Boost Vitamins 25%," *Drug Topics*, 12 Feb. 1940, p. 22.

45. Herman N. Bundesen, "The Mystic White Crystal of Health," *Ladies' Home Journal*, Feb. 1938, pp. 78, 80.

46. T. Swann Harding, "What about Vitamin Tablets?" *Scientific American*, May 1943, pp. 214–215.

47. "Vitamins Not for Colds," *Literary Digest*, 6 Feb. 1932, p. 27; Harding, "What about Vitamin Tablets?," pp. 214–215; Gaynor Maddox, "Vitamin Pills Are Not a Food Substitute," *Today's Health*, Nov. 1961, pp. 38, 74–76.

48. Linus Pauling, *Vitamin C and the Common Cold* (San Francisco: W. H. Freeman, 1970); "Vitamin C on the Cold Front: Cure or Craze?" *Senior Scholastic*, 8 Feb. 1971, p. 8.

49. A good source that summarizes much of the controversy in the first three years is Michael Halberstam, "The A, B-12, C, D and E of Vitamins," *New York Times Magazine*, 17 March 1974.

50. "Fla. Px Men Blame Vitamin C Shortage on Bad Weather and Nobel Scientist," *Drug Topics*, 21 Dec. 1970, p. 6; "Vitamin C Rush Hits Minn. Stores," *Drug Topics*, 15 Feb. 1971, p. 27. See also "A Warning on Vitamin C," *Newsweek*, 25 Jan. 1971, p. 90; "Gullible Skeptics: The Case of Vitamin C," *Science News*, 26 Dec. 1970, p. 477; Paul O'Neil, "The Vitamin C Mania," *Life*, 9 July 1971, pp. 55–56, 58–63.

51. "C: The Vitamin with Mystique," *Mademoiselle*, Nov. 1969, p. 189.

52. "Vitamin C, Anyone?" *Newsweek*, 30 Nov. 1970, pp. 62–64.

53. Doris Planz, "The Vitamin C Controversy," *Nation*, 5 April 1971, pp. 440–442.

54. "The Better Way: Can Vitamin C Really Prevent and Cure Colds?" *Good Housekeeping*, March 1971, pp. 173–175.

55. "Vitamin C—A Preventive of the Common Cold?" *Consumer Bulletin*, Sept. 1971, pp. 23–25.

56. J. M. Flagler, "You and the Big Vitamin Battle," *Look*, 1 June 1971, pp. 34–36, 40, 43.

57. Leticia Kent, "Dr. Linus Pauling Talks about Vitamin C and . . .," *Vogue*, 1 April 1971, p. 130.

58. O'Neil, "The Vitamin C Mania," pp. 55–56, 58–63; "C is for Controversy," *Newsweek*, 6 Dec. 1971, pp. 102–103.

59. Charles Glen King, "Warning: You Can Take Too Much Vitamin C," *McCall's*, March 1971, p. 65.

60. "Vitamin C—a Preventive of the Common Cold?," pp. 23–25.

61. Dodi Schultz, "The Verdict on Vitamins," *Today's Health*, Jan. 1974, pp. 54, 57–60, 63; Lowell Ponte, "The Facts about Vitamin C," *Reader's Digest*, Oct. 1980, pp. 94–97. See also Julie Wang, "Vitamin C: Dr. Pauling Was Right," *New York*, 9 April 1979, pp. 51, 53–54.

62. "New Findings about Vitamin C and the Common Cold," *Good Housekeeping*, April 1972, p. 201; "Vindicating Vitamin C," *Newsweek*, 21 Jan. 1974, p. 56.

63. "The Vitamins You Really Need," *Changing Times*, June 1974, pp. 18–20; "About the Furor over Vitamins," *U.S. News & World Report*, 15 July 1974, p. 63; Harold M. Schmeck, "2 Reports Find Little Merit in Using Vitamin C to Treat Colds," *New York Times*, 11 March 1975; Linus Pauling, "Letter to the Editor: Linus Pauling on Vitamin C," *New York Times*, 6 April 1975; Robert H. Morse, "Letter to the Editor: Pauling and Vitamin C: The 'Scrambled Facts,'" *New York Times*, 16 April 1975. For a detailed discussion of some of the major studies, see Kenneth J. Carpenter, *The History of Scurvy and Vitamin C* (Cambridge: Cambridge University Press, 1986), esp. pp. 210–220.

64. "Editorial: The Potency of Vitamin C," *Saturday Evening Post*, May 1974, p. 48.

65. Wang, "Vitamin C: Dr. Pauling Was Right"; Jane Stein, "Vitamins: How Much Is Too Much?" *McCall's*, Nov. 1979, pp. 129, 206, 208–210; "LHJ's Family Vitamin Chart," *Ladies Home Journal*, Dec. 1983, pp. 71–72; "Vitamins: How to Make Sure You Get What You Need," *McCall's*, Jan. 1985, pp. 48, 50, 52.

66. "Vitamins: How to Make Sure You Get What You Need"; Ponte, "The Facts about Vitamin C," pp. 94–97. See also Dianne Hales, "Vitamin C (as in Cure-All)," *Redbook*, March 1985, pp. 24, 26.

67. "As Vitamin Sales Pep up, So Do Worries on Overuse"; Council for Responsible Nutrition, "CRN 1993 Industry Data: Vitamin/Min Sales by Trade Class," *1993 Overview of the Nutritional Supplement Market*.

68. John C. Burnham, "American Medicine's Golden Age: What Happened to It?" in Judith Walzer Leavitt and Ronald L. Numbers, eds., *Sickness and Health in America: Readings in the History of Medicine and Public Health*, 2nd ed. (Madison: University of Wisconsin Press, 1985), pp. 248–258.

69. Joseph Bell, "The Facts and Myths about Vitamins," *Seventeen*, Aug. 1975, pp. 184–185, 215–216, 218. Bell also mentioned that opponents of Stare pointed out that in addition to his position at Harvard, the doctor was "connected with a large food processing company and that his heart [was] with the food industry," a relationship noted in few of the articles that quoted Stare.

## 4 THE HISTORY OF A VITAMIN DYNASTY

1. For more on the relationships between prescription companies and proprietary companies in the period, see Charles O. Jackson, *Food and Drug Legislation in the New Deal* (Princeton: Princeton University Press, 1970).
2. For the initial announcements in the trade press, see advertisement and "Miles Introduces Vitamin Tablets," *Drug Topics*, 28 Oct. 1940.
3. (Dr.) Elizabeth S. Lott, "Miles and Vitamins," typescript, located in the Miles Laboratories Archives, folder "Vitamins," undated (c. 1989).
4. Biographical information on Walter A. Compton comes from Lott, "Miles and Vitamins," ibid.; William C. Cray, *Miles, 1884–1984: A Centennial History* (Englewood Cliffs, N.J.: Prentice-Hall, 1984).
5. The Federal Trade Commission has jurisdiction over advertising; the Food and Drug Administration over labeling. At this time, labeling was defined to include not only labels on the bottles and tins, but also the packaging itself and any inserts. This was later extended to include any brochures and other publications displayed or sold with the product.
6. Cray, *Centennial History*, pp. 40–46.
7. Memorandum of interview, 12 Aug. 1940, attended by Dr. Walter Compton, Mr. Jack W. Clissold, Dr. E. M. Nelson, Mr. Ralph F. Kneeland, Jr., FDA Archives, Acc. no. 63A292, AF-13007.
8. Walter Compton to E. M. Nelson, 30 Aug. 1940; J. W. Clissold to E. M. Nelson, 2 Sept. 1940; G. P. Larrick to J. W. Clissold, 21 Sept. 1940; J. W. Clissold to G. P. Larrick, 24 Sept. 1940, all located in the FDA Archives, Acc. no. 63A292, AF-13007. For more on the FDA regulations, see chap. 6.
9. Larrick to Clissold, 5 Dec. 1940, located in the FDA Archives, Acc. no. 63A292.
10. Memorandum of interview, attended by Walter Compton, M. A. Rafferty, and Charles Beardsley (of Miles), and E. M. Nelson and R. F. Kneeland (of the FDA), 4 June 1941, FDA Archives, Acc. no. 63A292, AF-13007.
11. Ibid.
12. Larrick to Clissold, 5 Dec. 1940, FDA Archives, Acc. no. 63A292.
13. Attachment to letter from M. R. Stephens, chief of the St. Louis Station, FDA, to chief, Central District, 4 Feb. 1942, FDA Archives, Acc. no. 63A292, AF-13007.
14. M. R. Stephens to chief, Central District, 4 Feb. 1942; Chester T. Hubble to Commissioner of Food and Drugs, 6 Feb. 1942, FDA Archives, Acc. no. 63A292, AF-13007.
15. Miles Laboratories continued to consult with the FDA on new products and on changes in labeling and in the ingredients due to wartime restrictions. Memoranda and letters are on file in the FDA Archives, Acc. no. 63A292, AF-13007.
16. Lott, "Miles and Vitamins"; Cray, *Centennial History*, p. 58; "One-A-Day (Brand) Multiple Vitamins: History," undated typescript, Miles Laboratories Archives.

• • • • • • • • • • • • • • • • • • • • • • • • • • • • • • • • • • • • • • • •

17. See, for example, *Drug Topics*, 28 Oct. 1940, pp. 12–13; *Drug Topics*, 1 Dec. 1941, pp. 18–19; *Drug Topics*, 7 Jan. 1946, pp. 48–49.

18. W. H. Eddy, "How Many Vitamins a Day Do We Need?" *Good Housekeeping*, Jan. 1939, pp. 55, 85.

19. "One-A-Day" advertisement, *Parents' Magazine*, Dec. 1941, p. 80.

20. The concept of science often appeared in advertisements directed at women. They reinforced the development of the ideology of scientific motherhood, the belief that women needed contemporary scientific and medical advice to raise their children healthfully. For more on this point, see Rima D. Apple, "Constructing Mothers: Scientific Motherhood in the Nineteenth and Twentieth Centuries," *Social History of Medicine* 8 (1995): 161–178.

21. Cray, *Centennial History*, p. 58.

22. "Your Vitamins: An Important Subject Explained in Simple Terms the *One-A-Day* Way," Miles Laboratories, Inc., 1942, Miles Laboratories Archives.

23. Ibid., p. 3.

24. Cray, *Centennial History*, p. 58; "One-A-Day (Brand) Multiple Vitamins: History."

25. "Year 'Round: One-A-Day Vitamins for Your Whole Family," Miles Laboratories (1943).

26. Lott, "Miles and Vitamins."

27. F. L. McLaughlin, "One A Day (Brand) Vitamins: A History of Growth," typescript dated 10 Jan. 1961, Miles Laboratories Archives, folder "History."

28. Erwin Di Cyan and Stella Stakvel, "The Ubiquitous Vitamins Preparations," *Consumers' Research Bulletin*, Feb. 1944, pp. 5–9; March 1944, pp. 11–14.

29. R. M. Cunningham, Jr., "The Great Vitamin Scare," *The New Republic*, 26 Feb. 1945, pp. 287–290.

30. Ibid.; "Vimms Vanish," *Business Week*, 13 April 1946, pp. 102, 104.

31. Interview with Albert G. (Jeff) Wade II (October 1980), transcript in Miles Laboratories Archives.

32. "Minutes of Vitamin Conference, 26–27 May 1953," typescript in Walter A. Compton files, Miles Laboratories Archives.

33. "Vimms Vanish"; "Report of the Public Relations Committee," 10 Oct. 1961, typescript located in Walter A. Compton files, acc. no. 8301, Miles Laboratories Archives; "Food and Drug Businesses Gird for War over Vitamins, *New York Times*, 25 Aug. 1961.

34. "Vitamins and Your Health," New York: National Vitamin Foundation, 1964, Walter A. Compton files, acc. no. 8301, Miles Laboratories Archives.

35. "Vitamins and Your Health," New York: Vitamin Information Bureau, 1970, files concerning nutrition research and the FDA controversy, 1961–1970, acc. no. 8446a, Miles Laboratories Archives.

36. One-A-Day Plus Iron was announced in the trade press in early 1965, following a test-marketing in seven states. "Miles Labs Introduces New 'Vitamins-Plus-Iron,'" *Drug Topics*, 8 Feb. 1965, p. 56.

37. Interview with Albert G. (Jeff) Wade II (October 1980), transcript in Miles Laboratories Archives.

38. Letter from Frederick J. Cullen, M.D., medical consultant, to Dorothy Carter, M.D., 16 Dec. 1964, located in "One-A-Day Plus Iron Health Claims," Miles Laboratories Archives, acc. no. 8906, Legal Dept. Closed files.

39. Interoffice memorandum from Hugh A. Miller, M.D., "Use of Slogan 'For Better Health' in One-A-Day Multiple Vitamins and One-A-Day Plus Iron Advertising," 1 April 1965, located in "One-A-Day Plus Iron Health Claims," transcript, Miles Laboratories Archives, acc. no. 8906, Legal Dept. Closed files.

40. One-A-Day advertisement, *Drug Topics*, 10 Oct. 1960, pp. 34–35, reproduced this advertisement for the edification of druggists with the note explaining that this advertisement was designed to "give people a better understanding of the continuous importance of supplementary vitamins" and to help bring people into the pharmacy and, "at the same time, it can help to make your selling job easier."

41. "'Science' and Advertising: The Federal Trade Commission Is Seeking a Way to Curb Abuses," *Science*, 9 Dec. 1960, pp. 1749–1750.

42. "Extracts from a Marketing Research Department Report," 22 Jan. 1963, Walter A. Compton files, acc. no. 8301, Miles Laboratories Archives.

43. Interoffice memorandum, "Subject: Our One-A-Day Brand Vitamins," from Walter A. Compton to O. G. Kennedy, 23 Jan. 1963, Walter A. Compton files, acc. no. 8301, Miles Laboratories Archives.

44. Walter A. Compton to Frederick J. Cullen, 21 Jan. 1963, Walter A. Compton files, acc. no. 8301, Miles Laboratories Archives.

45. Interoffice memorandum, "Subject: Our One-A-Day brand vitamins," from Walter A. Compton to O. G. Kennedy, 23 Jan. 1963, Walter A. Compton files, acc. no. 8301, Miles Laboratories Archives.

46. Walter A. Compton to The Honorable Patrick V. McNamara, 24 Jan. 1963, copy in the Walter A. Compton files, acc. no. 8301, Miles Laboratories Archives.

47. Interoffice memorandum, from C. F. Miles to various Miles executives, including Compton, 31 Jan. 1963, Walter A. Compton files, acc. no. 8301, Miles Laboratories Archives.

48. See, for example, advertising copy for "Vitamins and You," prepared by Wade Advertising, Inc., 29 Jan. 1963, located in the Walter A. Compton files, acc. no. 8301, Miles Laboratories Archives.

49. Thomas R. A. Davis et al., "Review of Studies of Vitamin and Mineral Nutrition in the United States (1950–1968)," *Journal of Nutrition Education*, 1969, 1; file memorandum, from Joseph M. White, "Subject: Telephone conversation with Dr. Jean Mayer," 31 Oct. 1969, Walter A. Compton files, acc. no. 8301, Miles Laboratories Archives.

50. "Vitamins, Minerals and Americans," Miles Laboratories, Inc., 1970, copy in file concerning nutrition research and the FDA controversy, 1961–1970, acc. no. 8446a, Miles Laboratories Archives.

51. This point was proudly related by Compton in his testimony to the Senate Select Committee on Nutrition and Human Needs, 24 Feb. 1971, typescript

of summary statement located in "Nutrition-Health," acc. no. 8305, Miles Laboratories Archives.

52. Senate Select Committee on Nutrition and Human Needs, 24 Feb. 1971, typescript of summary statement located in "Nutrition-Health," acc. no. 8305, Miles Laboratories Archives; *Hearings before the U.S. Senate Select Committee on Nutrition and Human Needs: Part 1: Review of the Results of the White House Conference on Food, Nutrition, and Health* (Washington, D.C: Government Printing Office, 1972), pp. 197–259; *Part 10—Micronutrient Supplements for School Lunch Programs, 7 December 1971* (Washington, D.C.: Government Printing Office, 1972), pp. 2539–2620.

53. Press release, 20 June 1966, Miles Laboratories, Inc., Walter A. Compton files, acc. no. 8301, Miles Laboratories Archives. See also "Companies Study Food Proposals," *New York Times*, 24 July 1966; "Miles Answers FDA Regulations," *Drug Topics*, 25 July 1966, p. 56; Miles Laboratories, Inc., *Annual Report, 1966*, pp. 9–10.

54. Interoffice memorandum from Walter Roberts, Jr., to John Buckley, 15 July 1966, Walter A. Compton files, acc. no. 8301, Miles Laboratories Archives.

55. Press release, "Miles Opposes 'Deregulation' of Vitamin Supplements," 31 Oct. 1973, located in "News Releases, Notices, Announcements, 1971–1977," acc. no. 8322, Miles Laboratories Archives. See also form letter from Charles N. Jolly to congressional representatives, 18 May 1973, and "Summary Analysis and Position on 'The Food Supplement Amendment of 1973,'" both in the FDA History Office, file, "1976; Vitamin/Mineral Amend."

56. "Drug Firms Halt Children's TV Ads," *New York Times*, 21 July 1972. See also "Six Complaints Filed against Vitamin Ads," *CNI Weekly*, 1 June 1970, p. 6; "5 Weeks of Hearings Strengthen F.T.C.'s Determination to Continue Aggressive Regulation of TV Ads," *New York Times*, 22 Nov. 1971; "Senators Hear an Expert on TV Ads for Children," *New York Times*, 1 June 1972; Jay Arena, "Vitamin Pills and Children," *New York Times*, 30 June 1972; "Kids' Vitamin Ads Leave the Airwaves," *CNI Weekly*, 27 July 1972.

## 5 SCIENTIFIC EVIDENCE IN THE MARKETPLACE

1. There continues to be a lucrative market in today's world for acne medication—especially among teenagers, who can turn to a wide variety of over-the-counter and prescription drugs, hygienic rituals, dietary recommendations, and even their own support group, located in London: "Support Group Focuses on Acne," *Madison* (Wisc.) *Capital Times*, 24 June 1992. See also, Sharon Snider, "Acne: Taming That Age-Old Adolescent Affliction," *FDA Consumer*, October 1990.

2. Cohen & Aleshire, Inc., "Radio Continuity," 6 July 1961, Food and Drug Administration Archives, Record Group 88 (hereafter referred to as FDA RG88), AF-8-611. I wish to thank Dr. Suzanne White, FDA historian, for helping me locate these records.

3. 207 F.Supp. 758 (1962) (U.S. vs. Acnotabs and Pannett Products, Inc.); quotations are found on pp. 3–5.

4. For example, Ann-Shih Cheng, National Better Business Bureau, to Samuel L. Williams, Federal Trade Commission, 18 July 1960, FDA RG88, AF-8-611.

5. See FDA RG88, Acc. no. 66A 1030, box 70, for examples of consumers' letters on the subject of Acnotabs.

6. Gordon T. LaFlash to New York District Director, 19 Feb. 1960, located in FDA RG88, AF 8-611.

7. James Harvey Young, *The Medical Messiahs: A Social History of Health Quackery in Twentieth-Century America* (Princeton: Princeton University Press, 1967), pp. 206–208, 338–359.

8. Harry Milton Marks, "Regulating Medicine: The 1938 Drug Act," in *Ideas as Reforms: Therapeutic Experiments and Medical Practice, 1900–1980* (Ph.D. diss., Massschusetts Institute of Technology, 1987), pp. 51–91. See also Harry M. Marks, "Notes from the Underground: The Social Organization of Therapeutic Research," in Russell C. Maulitz and Diana E. Long, eds., *Grand Rounds: One Hundred Years of Internal Medicine* (Philadelphia: University of Pennsylvania Press, 1988), pp. 297–336; Abraham M. Lilienfeld, "*Ceteris Paribus*: The Evolution of the Clinical Trial," *Bulletin of the History of Medicine* 56 (1982): 1–18.

9. For more on the administrative power of the FDA, see Thomas H. Austern, "Sanctions in Silhouette: An Inquiry into the Enforcement of the Federal Food, Drug and Cosmetic Act," *Food Drug Cosmetic Law Journal*, Nov. 1963, pp. 617–631.

10. Post-Trial Memorandum, 9 July 1962, FDA RG88, Acc. no. 66A 1030, box 70, p. 29.

11. The description of the case is drawn from ibid.

12. Acnotabs was promoted as a combination of pancreatin, bile salts, pepsin, and vitamins A and C. It contained 10,000 IU of vitamin A. Even in the 1960s, when vitamin A was used in conjunction with other therapies in treating acne, it was prescribed in doses of 25,000 to 150,000 IU. Today, synthetic vitamin A is frequently prescribed in doses of 300,000 units.

13. Post-Trial Memorandum, 9 July 1962, FDA RG88, Acc. no. 66A 1030, box 70, pp. 22–23.

14. Ibid.

15. Ibid., pp. 24, 28.

16. Ibid., pp. 28–29.

17. Ibid., pp. 29–34.

18. Harry Milton Marks, "Historical Perspectives on Clinical Trials," working paper prepared for the National Research Council, unpublished manuscript, 1990. I am grateful to Prof. Marks for sharing this paper with me.

19. Post-Trial Memorandum, dated 9 July 1962, FDA RG88, Acc. no. 66A 1030, box 70, p. 10.

20. Ibid., pp. 41–42.

21. Ibid., p. 41.

22. Reply Brief prepared by the FDA, 20 July 1962, FDA RG88, Acc. no. 66A 1030, box 70, p. 10.

23. 207 F. Supp. 758 (1962), p. 13

24. Ibid., p. 16

25. Ibid., p. 17–18.

26. Letter from Goldhammer to Viault, 17 Aug. 1962; memo of interview, 4 Sept. 1962, FDA RG88, Acc. no. 66A 1030, box 70.

27. Ralph G. Smith, "Evaluation of Safety of New Drugs by the Food and Drug Administration," *Journal of New Drugs*, 1, 2 (1961): 59–64. Smith was director of the New Drug Branch, Bureau of Medicine, Food and Drug Administration.

28. Paul J. Quick, "Food and Drug Administration," in James Q. Wilson, ed., *The Politics of Regulation* (New York: Basic Books, 1980), pp. 197–198, citing FDA Commissioner George Larrick.

29. "Summary: Secretary Fleming's Meetings with Representatives of National Organizations, December 11, 17, and 18, 1958," typescript; "National Academy of Sciences—National Research Council: Report of Special Committee Advisory to the Secretary of Health, Education, and Welfare to Review the Policies, Procedures, and Decisions of the Division of Antibiotics and the New Drug Branch of the Food and Drug Administration," typescript; "Department of Health, Education, and Welfare: Staff Paper," prepared by the Food and Drug Administration, 1 Sept. 1960, typescript. All three documents are to be found in the FDA History Office files, Rockville, Md. I wish to thank Dr. John Swann, FDA historian, for his assistance in locating these reports.

30. Quoted in Peter Temin, *Taking Your Medicine: Drug Regulation in the United States* (Cambridge: Harvard Univ. Press, 1980), pp. 122–123.

31. Marks, "Historical Perspectives on Clinical Trials."

32. Kenneth G. Kohlstedt, "Developing and Testing of New Drugs by the Pharmaceutical Industry," *Journal of Clinical Pharmacology and Therapeutics* 1 (1960): 192–201.

33. Temin, *Taking Your Medicine*, pp. 123–124. See also Young, *Medical Messiahs*, pp. 413–422.

34. Quoted in Temin, *Taking Your Medicine*, p. 127. For contemporary analyses of this point, see Vincent A. Kleinfeld, "Recent Developments in Drug Labeling Regulations and Interpretations," *Publishing, Entertainment, Advertising and Allied Fields Law Quarterly* 4 (1964): 16–28; and "Drug Amendments of 1962: Federal Food, Drug, and Cosmetic Act," *Journal of New Drugs* 2 (1962): 314–320.

35. For an interesting comparative study of regulatory agencies' grappling with scientific claims, see Brendan Gillespie, Dave Eva, and Ron Johnston, "Carcinogenic Risk Assessment in the USA and UK: The Case of Aldrin/Dieldrin," in Barry Barnes and David Edge, eds., *Science in Context* (Cambridge: MIT Press, 1982), pp. 303–335.

36. Evelleen Richards analyzes an interesting example of this phenomenon

within the medical community in the case of Linus Pauling's advocacy of vitamin C in the treatment of cancer: *Vitamin C and Cancer: Medicine or Politics?* (New York: St. Martin's Press, 1991).

## 6 THE FDA AND CONSUMER PROTECTION

1. Peter Barton Hutt, "National Nutrition Policy and the Role of the Food and Drug Administration," *Currents: The Journal of Food, Nutrition & Health* 2, 2 (1986): 2–11.
2. "Vitamins Get a Book of Rules," *Business Week*, 6 April 1940, pp. 40–43.
3. "New Vitamin Rules," *Business Week*, 19 July 1941, p. 42.
4. Ruth and Edward Brecher, "Should You Take Vitamin Pills?" *Science Digest*, Oct. 1959, pp. 59–64; idem, "Are You Being Taken In by the 'Vitamin Racket'?" *Reader's Digest*, Nov. 1959, pp. 88–92.
5. See, for example, "Vitamins Get a Book of Rules"; Arthur W. Hafner et al., eds., *Guide to the American Medical Association Historical Health Fraud and Alternative Medicine Collection* (Chicago: American Medical Association, 1992).
6. Marjorie Hunter, "U.S. and A.M.A. Pledge Drive to End Billion-a-Year Quackery," *New York Times*, 7 Oct. 1961; James Harvey Young, "Nutritional Eccentricities," in *American Health Quackery* (Princeton: Princeton University Press, 1992), pp. 165–181.
7. U.S. Department of Health, Education and Welfare, Food and Drug Administration, news release, 20 June 1962 (copy in the FDA History Office, file, "1976: Vitamin/Mineral Amend."); "U.S. Acts to Curb Vitamin Labeling," *New York Times*, 20 June 1962.
8. Similar to the standards of identity promoted for food products, the 1962 standards were designed to "promote honest and fair dealing for the consumer." Dr. Suzanne White, FDA historian, personal communication, 7 June 1994. See also Suzanne Rebecca White, "Chemistry and Controversy: Regulating the Use of Chemicals in Foods, 1883–1959" (Ph.D. diss., Emory University, 1994).
9. Alfred E. Harper, "Nutritional Regulations and Legislation—Past Developments, Future Implications, *Journal of the American Dietetic Association* 71 (Dec. 1977): 601–609; Harold M. Schmeck, Jr., "U.S. Stiffens Rules on Dietetic Foods, *New York Times*, 18 June 1966. More about the National Health Federation can be found in Young, "Nutritional Eccentricities."
10. William M. Carley, "FDA Move to Restrict Ingredients of Vitamin Compounds Is Imminent," *Wall Street Journal*, 10 June 1966. See, for example, U.S. Department of Health, Education and Welfare, Food and Drug Administration, Student Reference Sheet, "Health Education vs. Medical Quackery," SR-13 (1966) (copy located in the University of Wisconsin Pharmacy Library, Kremer Reference Files, C46 [g] III [i]); U.S. Department of Health, Education and Welfare, Food and Drug Administration, "Your Money and Your Life: An FDA Catalog of Fakes and Swindles in the Health Field," FDA Publication no. 19, Oct. 1963 (copy located in the University of Wisconsin Pharmacy Library, Kremer Reference Files, C46 [g] III [i]).

11. See, for example, "Should the Government Tell *You* What Vitamins to Take? *Truth* 3, 3 (1964): 10–17.

12. Schmeck, "U.S. Stiffens Rules on Dietetic Foods"; "Nutrition: Vitamin Crackdown," *Time*, 1 July 1966, pp. 48–49. Crepe labels had been used in the food industry. The canning industry helped push through the 1930 McNary-Mapes Amendment to the 1906 Food and Drug Act. This amendment permitted the establishment of standards for all canned foods, except meats and milk. Items not meeting the standards displayed a crepe label to identify the product as "below U.S. Standard, low quality, but not illegal." White, "Chemistry and Controversy," p. 259.

13. Ralph Lee Smith, "Showdown on Vitamins," *Nation*, 28 Nov. 1966, pp. 578–580.

14. Ibid.

15. James J. Nagel, "Companies Study Food Proposals," *New York Times*, 24 July 1996.

16. "12 Drug Companies File Suit to Prevent New Controls," *New York Times*, 22 Sept. 1966.

17. "F.D.A. Orders Delay in Diet Regulations," *New York Times*, 15 Dec. 1966.

18. U.S. Department of Health, Education and Welfare, Food and Drug Administration, "FDA Fact Sheet: Special Dietary Regulations," (1967) (copy in the University of Wisconsin Pharmacy Library, Kremer Reference Files, C46 [g] III [i]–1967).

19. U.S. Department of Health, Education and Welfare, Food and Drug Administration, "FDA News Release," 1 April 1968 (copy in the University of Wisconsin Pharmacy Library, Kremer Reference File, C46 [g] III [i] U.S., National 1968).

20. "Vitamin Hearings to Discuss Labels," *New York Times*, 19 May 1968.

21. Kirkpatrick W. Dilling to the FDA, 1 June 1967, FDA Archives, Acc. no. 88-75-3, o51.18.

22. Frederick J. Stare to Herbert Ley, 1 July 1968, FDA Archives, Acc. no. 88-75-3, o51.18.

23. Other letters preserved in the files are from Harold E. Harrison, M.D., Baltimore City Hospitals; Bacon F. Chow, professor of biochemistry, Johns Hopkins School of Hygiene and Public Health; W. N. Pearson, professor of biochemistry, Vanderbilt University; George M. Owen, M.D., professor of pediatrics, Ohio State University; and Paul György, among others.

24. L. J. Filer, M.D., to Herbert Ley, 4 Nov. 1968, FDA Archives, Acc. no. 88-76-80, o51.18.

25. Calvin Woodruff to Herbert Ley, 2 Oct. 1968, FDA Archives, Acc. no. 88-76-80, o51.18.

26. Herbert Ley to Robert S. Harris, 7 Oct. 1968, FDA Archives, Acc. no. 88-76-80, o51.18.

27. Herbert Ley to Frederick J. Stare, 23 July 1968, FDA Archives, Acc. no. 88-76-80, o51.18.

28. "Vitamin Hearings to Discuss Labels," *New York Times*, 19 May 1968.

29. J. I. Rodale, "Who Needs Food Supplements?" *Organic Gardening and Farming* (Aug. 1968): 83–87.

30. James S. Turner, *The Chemical Feast: The Ralph Nader Study Group on Food Protection and the Food and Drug Administration* (New York: Grossman, 1970), p. 209.

31. Quoted in ibid., pp. 41–42.

32. Ibid., p. 72.

33. Philip M. Boffey, "Nader's Raiders on the FDA: Science and Scientists 'Misused,'" *Science*, 17 April 1970, 349–352. A copy of "Objections of Sebrell, Chairman of Food & Nutrition Board Cmte. on Dietary Allowance" is located in the Miles Laboratories Archives, Walter A. Compton files, box 5, folder, "FDA vitamin regulations." See also memo from William H. Sumerson, Director of Bureau of Science, to James L. Goddard, Commission of Food and Drugs, Subject: Conference with Dr. Henry Sebrell, 4 April 1967, FDA Archives, Acc. no. 88-75-3. Though the FDA representatives concluded that "the 'apparent' controversy fostered by the Trade Press between the Food and Nutrition Board and FDA appears to be no more than a distorted interpretation of the situation," it is just such an "interpretation" that demonstrated the fragility of scientific consensus in nutritional science over vitamin usage. For more on the history of RDAs, see A. E. Harper, "Origin of Recommended Dietary Allowances—An Historic Overview," *American Journal of Clinical Nutrition* 41 (1985): 140–148.

34. "Vitamin C—A Preventive of the Common Cold?" *Consumer Bulletin*, Sept. 1971, p. 23.

35. J. M. Flagler, "You and the Big Vitamin Battle: Millions Swear by Vitamins, Yet Experts Disagree. Who Wins and Who Loses?" *Look*, 1 June 1971, pp. 34–36, 40, 43.

36. The Pharmaceutical Manufacturers Association released daily reports on hearings. A collection of these newsletters many be found in the Miles Laboratories Archives, Acc. no. 8446a—Files concerning Nutrition Research and the FDA Vitamin labeling controversy, 1961–1970, box 2, folder, "Daily reports on drug hearing."

37. Schmeck, "U.S. Stiffens Rules on Dietetic Foods."

38. "After Years of Dispute: Stricter Controls on Vitamins," *U.S. News & World Report*, 13 Aug. 1973, p. 83.

39. Harold M. Schmeck, Jr., "Vitamin Sales and Labeling Face Tighter Regulation by the F.D.A.," *New York Times*, 2 Aug. 1973.

40. Marlene Cimons, "New Vitamin Rules: Rx for Consumer?" *Newsday*, 26 April 1973.

41. "The FDA Fights the Vitamin Craze," *Business Week*, 15 July 1972, p. 28.

42. Ibid.

43. "Major Retiree Group Endorses New FDA Vitamin Regulations," news release of the National Retired Teachers Association–American Association of Retired Persons (1973), the University of Wisconsin Pharmacy Library, Kremer Reference Files, C46 (g) III (i)–1973.

44. "After Years of Dispute," p. 83.

45. Form letter signed by Anita Johnson for the Health Research Group, c. May 1973, FDA History Office, file, "1976: Vitamin/Mineral Amend."

46. U.S. House of Representatives, *Hearings before the Subcommittee on Public Health and Environment, Committee on Interstate and Foreign Commerce*, 29–31 Oct. 1973, 93rd Cong., p. 614.

47. For an interesting analysis of the importance and use of "ignorance claims" among scientists and journalists, see S. Holly Stocking and Lisa W. Holstein, "Constructing and Reconstructing Scientific Ignorance," *Knowledge: Creation, Diffusion, Utilization* 15 (December 1993): 186–210. They explain: "Scientists make claims that something is not known (because existing knowledge is absent, incomplete, uncertain, distorted, irrelevant, or otherwise limited) and so not useful, and they offer these claims in ways that reflect, protect, and advance their interests" (p. 205).

## 7  SCIENCE IN CONSUMER POLITICS

1. Harold M. Schmeck, Jr., "Vitamin Sales and Labeling Face Tighter Regulation by the F.D.A.," *New York Times*, 2 Aug. 1973.

2. There are many examples of these petitions in the FDA Archives, Acc. no. 88-75-3, o51.18.

3. Letter from M. R., 6 Dec. 1966, FDA Archives, Acc. no. 88-75-3, o51.18.

4. Letter from L.A.D., 7 Nov. 1969, FDA Archives, Acc. no. 88-76-80, o51.18. Emphasis in original.

5. Correspondence between Raymond Chen and Schmidt, 2 Jan. 1974 and 14 Jan. 1974, FDA Archives, Acc. no. 88-80-17, o51.18.

6. Letter from R.M.H., 10 Oct. 1972, FDA Archives, Acc. no. 88-78-19, o51.18.

7. Letter from N. (Mrs. W. A.) B., 15 Oct. 1972, FDA Archives, Acc. no. 88-78-19, o51.18.

8. Ibid.

9. Letter from Mrs. F. S., 22 Sept. 1972, FDA Archives, Acc. no. 88-78-19, o51.18.

10. Letter from "A concerned American," Mrs. D.E.M., 18 Dec. 1972, FDA Archives, Acc. no. 88-79-23, o51.18.

11. Alfred E. Harper, "Nutritional Regulations and Legislation—Past Developments, Future Implications," *Journal of the American Dietetic Association*, 71, 6 (Dec. 1977): 601–609.

12. For more on the controversies over the nutritional changes in American food due to the processing industry, see Warren J. Belasco, *Appetite for Change: How the Counterculture Took on the Food Industry, 1966–1988* (New York: Pantheon, 1989).

13. Suzanne Rebecca White, "Chemistry and Controversy: Regulating the Uses of Chemicals in Foods, 1883–1959" (Ph.D. diss., Emory University, 1994), pp. 263–265, 309–361.

14. Letter from "A concerned American," Mrs. D.E.M., 18 Dec. 1972, FDA Archives, Acc. no. 88-79-23, o51.18.

15. Letter from S. U., [7 Oct. 1972?], FDA Archives, Acc. no. 88-78-19, o51.18.
16. Letter from T.E.C., 30 Oct. 1972, FDA Archives, Acc. no. 88-78-19, o51.18.
17. Letter from A.M.H., 5 Nov. 1972, FDA Archives, Acc. no. 88-78-19, o51.18.
18. Letter from V. D., 14 Dec. 1972, FDA Archives, Acc. no. 88-78-23, o51.18.
19. Letter from C.R.H., Oct. 1972, FDA Archives, Acc. no. 88-78-19, o51.18.
20. Jeanne Mangels, FDA Office of Consumer Inquiries, 22 Nov. 1972, responding to a letter from A.M.H., FDA Archives, Acc. no. 88-78-19, o51.18.
21. Letter from Gerald F. Meyer to M. McB., 16 Nov. 1972, FDA Archives, Acc. no. 88-78-19, o51.18.
22. Letter from T. H., 7 Aug. 1973, FDA Archives, Acc. no. 88-79-23, o51.18.
23. Letter from W.R.M., 3 March 1973, FDA Archives, Acc. no. 88-79-23, o51.18.
24. Letter from M. S., 20 Aug. 1973, FDA Archives, Acc. no. 88-79-23, o51.18.
25. Letter from H.S.F., 31 May 1973, FDA Archives, Acc. no. 88-79-23, o51.18.
26. Letter from Peter Barton Hutt, Assistant General Counsel, FDA, to M.A.S., 10 Sept. 1973, FDA Archives, Acc. no. 88-79-23, o51.18.
27. Letter from William E. Braunig, Consumer Safety Officer, Office of Legislative Services, FDA, to B.L.G., 24 Aug. 1973, FDA Archives, Acc. no. 88-79-23, o51.18.
28. Letter from C. A., 16 Feb. 1973, FDA Archives, Acc. no. 88-79-23, o51.18.
29. Letter from R. D., 3 Aug. 1973, FDA Archives, Acc. no. 88-79-23, o51.18.
30. Letter from F. M., 5 Aug. 1973, FDA Archives, Acc. no. 88-79-23, 051.18.
31. Letter from H.S.F., 31 May 1973, FDA Archives, Acc. no. 88-79-23, o51.18.

## 8 VITAMINS IN THE POLITICAL PROCESS

1. John J. Fried, *The Vitamin Conspiracy* (New York: Saturday Review Press, E.P. Dutton, 1975), pp. 16–18.
2. U.S. House of Representatives, *Hearings before the Subcommittee on Public Health and Environment, Committee on Interstate and Foreign Commerce*, 93rd Congress, 29–31 Oct. 1973 [hereafter referred to as House hearings], pp. 302, 776; Nicholas von Hoffman, "Of Excess and Exorcism," *Washington Post*, 11 June 1973.
3. House hearings, pp. 39–48, 175–176, 196.
4. Richard D. Lyons, "Disputed Health Lobby is Pressing for a Bill to Overturn Any Limits on Sales of Vitamins," *New York Times*, 14 May 1973.
5. House hearings: see, for example, testimony of C. E. Butterwork, Jr., p. 625; Charles N. Jolly, p. 645; Stanley N. Gershoff, p. 572; and Joseph M. Wile, p. 644.
6. Ibid., Charles N. Jolly, pp. 645–659. See also Stanley N. Gershoff, pp. 665, 673; Cyril F. Brickfield, pp. 223–225.
7. Ibid., William R. Roy, p. 446.
8. Ibid., Claude Pepper, p. 752.
9. Ibid., Herman W. Dorn, p. 458.
10. Ibid., Roger J. Williams, p. 313.
11. Ibid., Ruth Desmond, p. 264.

12. Ibid., William Randall, p. 602.
13. Ibid., B. F. Sick, p. 732; Bill Archer, p. 783; John Melcher, p. 777. Through much of this controversy, most participants drew a line between vitamins with little or no toxicity, such as water soluble vitamin C, and those of known toxicity, such as fat soluble vitamins A and D. The underlying assumption for even the most vocal vitamin supporters was that the FDA would continue to regulate harmful substances.
14. Ibid., Wendell Wyatt, p. 755.
15. Ibid., John A. Blatnik, pp. 727–728.
16. Nancy L. Ross, "Battle of the ABCs," *Washington Post*, 15 Aug. 1974.
17. House hearings, Mrs. Lee Aitkin, p. 281.
18. William Claiborne, "Coalition Beats Back Curb on Vitamin Pills," *Washington Post*, 22 Aug. 1974.
19. For much of the data in this section I am indebted to Howard E. Shuman, interview on 5 Nov. 1993. Shuman was administrative assistant to Senator Proxmire from 1969 to 1982.
20. William Proxmire, *Uncle Sam—Last of the Big-Time Spenders* (New York: Simon and Schuster, 1972), p. 221.
21. William Proxmire, *You Can Do It! Senator Proxmire's Exercise, Diet and Relaxation Plan* (New York: Simon and Schuster, 1973), pp. 181–185. The book received wide press coverage. Helen Anderson, "Patriotic Duty to Get in Shape: Proxmire," *Oshkosh Daily*, 5 Sept. 1973; Jim Kornkven, "Proxmire Claims You Can Do It!," *Kenosha Evening News*, 11 Sept. 1973; Marian Christy, "Proxmire: Just for the Health of It," *Boston Sunday Globe*, 2 Dec. 1973, all located in the William Proxmire Papers, M78-602, State Historical Society of Wisconsin Archives.
22. Shuman interview.
23. Letter from E.W.M., to William Proxmire, 20 Sept. 1974, FDA Archives, Acc. no. 88-80-17, o51.18.
24. Shuman interview.
25. *Congressional Record—Senate*, 12 Dec. 1973, 40939–40946.
26. Ibid., 10 June 1974, 18477–18478.
27. Rosemary Kendrick, "Vitamins Not Drugs: Prox Bill Passes," *Madison* (Wisc.) *Capital Times*, 12 Dec. 1975.
28. William Claiborne, "Coalition Beats Back Curb on Vitamin Pills," *Washington Post*, 22 Aug. 1974; "FDA Controls on Vitamin Hit in Senate," *Washington Post*, 15 Aug. 1974.
29. U.S. Senate, *Hearings before the Subcommittee on Public Health, Committee on Labor and Public Welfare*, 93rd Congress, 14 and 22 Aug. 1974 [hereafter referred to as Senate hearings], William Proxmire, p. 873.
30. Ibid., William Proxmire, pp. 12–15.
31. Ibid., C. E. Butterworth, pp. 546–547; Alvin M. Mauer, p. 560; M. Daniel Tatkon, p. 903.
32. Ibid., Alexander Schmidt, pp. 342–343, 523–524. The exchange between

• • • • • • • • • • • • • • • • • • • • • • • • • • • • • • • • • • • • • •

Proxmire and Schmidt was also reported in "F.D.A. Vitamin Curbs Scorned by Proxmire," *New York Times*, 15 Aug. 1974.

33. Senate hearings, Victor Herbert, p. 677. See also "The Massive Vitamin Dose Dispute: The Next Move Is Congress'," *Medical World News*, 13 Jan. 1975, pp. 95, 99, 100, 103. Herbert defines himself as a "quackbuster." A recent news article described Herbert's objections to the display of a book entitled *Alternative Medicine: A Guide* at the Ellis Island immigration museum. The museum closed the exhibit containing the book and had pulled the book from its bookstore. The museum is now enmeshed in a swirl of controversy and faces a lawsuit from the book's publisher. Herbert, however, is confident in his position and denies any dispute, declaring: "There's no controversy. It's a quack book. I'm a scientist. I only state facts. I don't give opinions." James Barron, "Professor Battles Ellis Island Exhibit," *New York Times*, 25 Aug. 1994.

34. "Massive Vitamin Dose Dispute," pp. 95, 99, 100, 103.

35. Senate hearings, M. Daniel Tatkon, p. 905.

36. "Rules on Vitamins Put Off 6 Months," *New York Times*, 17 Aug. 1974; Claiborne, "Coalition Beats Back Curb on Vitamin Pills"; "Supreme Court Upholds FDA Vitamin Authority," *CNI Weekly Report*, 6 March 1975, p. 8.

37. David Burnham, "F.D.A. Eases Rules on Some Vitamins," *New York Times*, 28 May 1975.

38. "FDA Proposed New Vitamin Regs," *CNI Weekly Report*, 26 June 1975, p. 6.

39. Burnham, "F.D.A. Eases Rules on Some Vitamins."

40. *Congressional Record—Senate*, 17 Sept. 1974, pp. 31368–31369; 24 Sept. 1974, pp. 32333–32337, 32376; 8 May 1975, pp. 13508–13510; 15 July 1975, pp. 22778–22780.

41. Press release, "Proxmire, Schweiker Offer Vitamin Bill," 3 Feb. 1975, located in the Proxmire Papers, M88-133, State Historical Society of Wisconsin Archives.

42. Kendrick, "Vitamins Not Drugs: Prox Bill Passes."

43. Public Law 94-278, 94th Congress, H.R. 7988, 22 April 1976. The legislative chronology can be traced through "FDA Vitamin Regulations: Should They Be Overturned?" *Congressional Quarterly Weekly Report*, 12 Jan. 1974, pp. 63–66; "Vitamin Regulations," *Congressional Quarterly Weekly Report*, 24 Aug. 1974, pp. 2276; "Vitamin Rider," *Congressional Quarterly Weekly Report*, 28 Sept. 1974, p. 2638; "Vitamins," *Congressional Quarterly Weekly Report*, 20 Dec. 1975, p. 2783; "Vitamin Regulation," *Congressional Quarterly Weekly Report*, 17 April 1976.

44. James Harvey Young, "Nutritional Eccentricities," in *American Health Quackery* (Princeton: Princeton University Press, 1992), p. 175.

45. Harold Hopkins, "Regulating Vitamins and Minerals," *FDA Consumer*, July–August 1976, pp. 10–11.

46. See, for example, Arielle Emmett, "Are You Overdosing on Vitamins? The ABC & D of Vitamin Lore," *Ms.*, April 1978, pp. 13–14, 16, 20; Connie Bruck, "Vitamins," *New Times*, 24 July 1978, pp. 54–56, 58–62; Mary-Ellen Banashek, "Vitamins: What to Know before You Decide You Need Them," *Mademoiselle*, August 1978, pp. 217, 278.

47. Committee quote is found in Steven Findlay, "Latest Dispatch from the Vitamin Front," *U.S. News & World Report,* 6 Nov. 1989, pp. 100–101; Richard L. Worsnop, "Dietary Supplements," *CQ Researcher,* 8 July 1994, pp. 577–599. See also Karen Glenn, "How to Get the Most from Your Vitamins," *McCall's,* Feb. 1986, pp. 73–74, 76, 79–80; "Vitamins: When More Is Too Much," *Changing Times,* April 1986, pp. 45–49.

48. For instructions on how to set up for Blackout Day, see the "Dietary Supplement Blackout Kit" prepared by the National Nutritional Foods Association. I thank Cheryl Hughes of the Whole Wheatery, Lancaster, Calif., for supplying me with a copy of the kit and other materials distributed by the National Nutritional Foods Association, the National Health Alliance, and the Citizens for Health.

49. Miriam Shuchman and Michael Wilkes, "The Vitamin Uprising," *New York Times Magazine,* 2 Oct. 1994, pp. 79, 87–89.

50. Julie Rovner, "New FDA 'User Fee' Bill Clears; Vitamin Labeling Addressed," *Congressional Quarterly Weekly Report,* 10 Oct. 1992, p. 3169.

51. "Vitamin Rules May Become Weaker," *Madison* (Wisc.) *Capital Times,* 11 May 1994. See also Roy Upton, "Shotgun Regulating: Will Dietary Supplements Become Prescription 'Drugs'?" *E: The environmental magazine,* September 1992, pp. 52–53.

52. Orrin G. Hatch, "Congress versus the Food and Drug Administration: How One Government Health Agency Harms the Public Health," *Journal of Public Policy and Marketing* 13 (Spring 1994): 151–152.

53. Bruce Silverglade, "The Vitamin Wars—Marketing, Lobbying, and the Consumer," *Journal of Public Policy and Marketing* 13 (Spring 1994): 152–154.

54. Worsnop, "Dietary Supplements," p. 580.

55. "Gains in the Vitamin War," *New York Times,* 20 Oct. 1994.

## CONCLUSION

1. Dan Rennick, "Vitamin Volume Totaled $179,850,000 in 1943," *Drug Topics,* 29 May 1944, p. 43; "Pharmacy Gets Bigger Share of Vitamin Volume," *Drug Topics,* 9 July 1945, p. 55.

2. "Vitamins & Toys Yield High Volume on Fount Backbar," *Drug Topics,* 10 Oct. 1960, p. 90; "Vitamins Sell When They Are Seen, *Drug Topics,* 22 Aug. 1966, p. 47.

3. "Vitamin Gifts Attract 1500 Youngsters on Halloween," *Drug Topics,* 7 Oct. 1963, p. 76.

4. Jane Stein, "Vitamins: How Much Is Too Much? *McCall's,* Nov. 1979, p. 129. See also "Vitamin Group Says Many Americans Are Nutritionally Below Average," *Drug Topics,* 22 Aug. 1966, pp. 2, 30; B.A.S, "Vitamins: Dispelling the Myths," *Forecast for Home Economics,* March 1979, p. 38; Emily Greenspan, "Vitamins: Do You Really Need a Daily Dose?" *Mademoiselle,* April 1983, pp. 147–149, 282–283.

5. Blossom H. Patterson et al., "Fruit and Vegetables in the American Diet:

Data from the NHANES II Survey," *American Journal of Public Health* 80 (1990): 1443–1449; Jube Shiver, "As Vitamin Sales Pep Up, So Do Worries on Overuse," *Los Angeles Times*, 23 March 1986. See also Anastasia Toufexis, "The New Scoop on Vitamins," *Time*, 6 April 1992, pp. 54–59 (abridged and reprinted in *Reader's Digest*, August 1992, pp. 86–90); Mirka Knaster, "The New Power of Vitamins: Can Supplements Help Boost Immunity and Prevent Disease? A Lot More Doctors Now Say Yes," *Ladies' Home Journal*, Aug. 1992, pp. 94, 96, 98–99.

6. Jud Carrol, "Vitamins Go Multiple," *Druggists Circular*, March 1939, 22–23, 82, 87, 90.

7. Paul de Kruif, "How to Prolong the Prime of Life," *Reader's Digest*, June 1957, pp. 139–42. See also "Don't Overdo on Vitamins," *Changing Times*, Feb. 1957, pp. 23–24.

8. *Operation Petticoat*, directed by Blake Edwards, 1959.

9. Greg Howard, "Sally Forth," syndicated cartoon, 1 Dec. 1993.

10. Rite Aero and Stephanie Rick, *Vitamin Power: A User's Guide to Nutritional Supplements & Botanical Substances That Can Change Your Life* (New York: Harmony Books, 1987).

11. *Globe*, 16 Oct. 1990.

12. Natalie Angier, *New York Times*, 10 March 1992; Scott Russell, *Madison* (Wisc.) *Capital Times*, 1 Feb. 1994.

13. Toufexis, "New Scoop on Vitamins."

14. See, for example, Knaster, "New Power of Vitamins"; Diane Debrovner, "Do You Really Need Vitamins?" *McCalls*, April 1992, p. 38; Mary Ann Howkins, "The Big Vitamin Debate," *Glamour*, August 1994, pp. 204–207; Geoffrey Cowley and Vernon Church, "Live Longer with Vitamin C: A New Study Finds That a Little More Is a Lot Better," *Newsweek*, 18 May 1992, p. 60; Geoffrey Cowley, "Vitamin Revolution," *Newsweek*, 7 June 1993, pp. 46–49; Lawrence E. Altman, "Vitamin Array Is Found to Be Benefit to Elderly," *New York Times*, 6 Nov. 1992; Carol Gentry, "MDs Rethinking Vitamins," *Chicago Tribune*, 15 Jan. 1993.

15. Bonnie Liebman and David Schardt, "Vitamin Smarts," *Nutrition Action*, Nov. 1995, p. 1; "The Supplement-Takers Guide to the Universe," *Nutrition Action*, Jan.-Feb. 1993; "A 9-Point Guide to Choosing the Right Supplement," *Tufts University Diet and Nutrition Letter*, Sept. 1993.

16. Gentry, "MDs Rethinking Vitamins."

17. Cowley, "Vitamin Revolution."

18. Physicians Plus, "Facts about Vitamin-Mineral Supplements," Madison, Wisc.: Feb. 1992.

19. Gina Kolata, "Vitamin Supplements Are Seen as No Guard against Diseases," *New York Times*, 14 April 1994; Geoffrey Cowley, "Are Supplements Still Worth Taking?" *Newsweek*, 25 April 1994, p. 47; Mary Ann Howkins, "The Big Vitamin Debate," *Glamour*, Aug. 1994, pp. 204–207.

20. Buring quoted in Howkins, "Big Vitamin Debate." See also "Taking Vitamins: Can They Prevent Disease?" *Consumer Reports*, Sept. 1994, pp. 563–564.

21. "The Vitamin Pushers," *Consumer Reports*, March 1986, pp. 170–175. The earliest piece on vitamins to appear in *CR* was Walter C. Alvarez, "The Vitamin Stampede," *Consumer Reports*, Dec. 1936, pp. 23–24, in which Alvarez, a Mayo Clinic physician, decried the overselling of vitamins. The next broad-based vitamin article in *CR* was "The Facts about Vitamins," Sept. 1960, pp. 493–496, followed by "More of the Facts You Should Know about Vitamins," Jan. 1961, pp. 44–48, which sought to answer readers' objections to the content of the previous article. Consistent through these and also various editions of CU's book *The Medicine Show* (subtitled *Some Plain Truths about Popular Products for Common Ailments* in editions published in 1961, 1963, 1970, 1974, and 1980) were that vitamin supplementation was unnecessary, that all the required micronutrients were available in a well-balanced diet, that there was no such thing as subclinical deficiency, and that the industry was overselling its products.

22. "Vitamin Pushers," Technical Check Copy, the Consumers Union Archives, folder "The Vitamin Pushers, March 1986, pp. 170–175."

23. Galleys dated 19 Jan. 1986, Consumers Union Archives, folder, "The Vitamin Pushers, March 1986, pp. 170–175."

24. Draft dated 13 Jan. 1986, composite marked up typescript also dated 13 Jan. Galleys dated 19 Jan. and page proofs dated 24 Jan. 1986, Consumers Union Archives, folder, "The Vitamin Pushers, March 1986, pp. 170–175."

25. J.W.E. to CU, 14 Feb. 1986, Consumers Union Archives, folder, "Vitamins."

26. M.T. to CU, 14 April 1986, Consumers Union Archives, folder, "Vitamins."

27. H.R.P., Jr., to CU, 8 March 1986, Consumers Union Archives, folder, "Vitamins."

28. "Can You Live Longer? What Works and What Doesn't," *Consumer Reports*, Jan. 1992, pp. 7–15.

29. "The Supplement Story: Can Vitamins Help?" *Consumer Reports*, Jan. 1992, pp. 12–13.

30. Marked-up copy of typescript of "Can vitamins help?," located in the Consumers Union Archives, folder, "Can You Live Longer? Jan. 1992, p. 7–15."

31. "The Supplement Story," pp. 13, 12.

32. "Taking Vitamins: Can They Prevent Disease?" *Consumer Reports*, Sept. 1994, pp. 561–564.

33. Ibid., pp. 561–562.

34. "Buying Vitamins: What's Worth the Price? *Consumer Reports*, Sept. 1994, pp. 564–569.

35. Ernest Dichter, "A Psychological Research Study of the Sales and Advertising Problems of One A Day," Institute for Research in Mass Motivations, Inc., Dec. 1953, submitted to Miles Laboratories, Miles Archives, Acc. no. 8343—Consumer Products Studies and Statements, 1939–1973, box 3.

36. "Vitamin Survey: A *Good Housekeeping* Consumer Panel Report," 1958.

37. "Development and Testing of Vitamin Concepts: A Report Based on Three Waves of Qualitative Interviews on Vitamin Concepts," prepared for Miles Laboratories, Feb. 1964, Miles Archives Acc. no. 8341, Records of the Con-

• • • • • • • • • • • • • • • • • • • • • • • • • • • • • • • • • • • • • • • • •

sumer Products/Marketing Research Dept., box 10, folder, "Prod. Vitamins—Studies-Markets."

38. The data for the next paragraphs have been drawn from National Analysts, Inc., *A Study of Health Practices and Opinions,* conducted for the Food and Drug Administration, Department of Health, Education and Welfare, June 1972; Response Analysis Corp., "Food and Nutrition: Knowledge, Beliefs," a nationwide study among food shoppers for the Division of Consumer Studies, Bureau of Foods, Food and Drug Administration, March 1974; "Vitamin issues," 3, 2 (July 1984) (publication of the Vitamin Nutrition Information Service of Hoffmann-La Roche); Mary M. Bender et al., "Trends in Prevalence and Magnitude of Vitamin and Mineral Supplement Usage and Correlation with Health Status," *Journal of the American Dietetic Association* 92 (1992): 1096–1101; "Vitamin Usage in the United States," June 1991, the Vitamin Nutrition Information Service of Hoffmann-La Roche; Council for Responsible Nutrition, *1993 Overview of the Nutritional Supplement Market* (Washington, D.C.: CRN, 1994). Reports of these findings were repeated frequently in the popular press, sometimes with attributions, often not. See, for example, J. M. Flagler, "You and the Big Vitamin Battle: Millions Swear by Vitamins, Yet Experts Disagree: Who Wins and Who Loses?" *Look,* 1 June 1971, pp. 34–36, 40, 34; "FDA Vitamin Regulations under Attack in Congress," *Consumer Reports,* June 1975, pp. 337–338; Lewis Vaughn, "Who Takes Vitamins?" *Prevention Magazine,* Feb. 1984, pp. 22–25.

39. *Study of Health Practices,* Part 1, p. 9; Part 2, p. 7; part 2, p. 12.

40. Ibid., "Summary and Conclusions," p. iii; "Chapter 1: Introduction," p. 1.

41. Dorothy Phillips, "Catering to the 'Take-Charge' Consumer," *Marketing Communications,* Nov. 1985, pp. 23–31.

42. Bender et al., "Trends"; "Vitamin usage in the United States"; Vaughn, "Who Takes Vitamins?"; Janet T. McDonald, "Vitamin and Mineral Supplement Use in the United States," *Clinical Nutrition,* Jan.-Feb. 1986, pp. 27–33.

43. Eugenia C. English and Jennifer W. Carl, "Use of Nutritional Supplements by Family Practice Patients," *JAMA,* 11 December 1981, pp. 2719–2721. See also Kathi Gannon, "Americans Often Don't Have Facts about the Vitamins They Take," *Drug Topics,* 6 Aug. 1990, pp. 24, 26.

44. See, for example, Joe Graedon, "The Vitamin Dilemma," *Medical Self-Care,* Spring 1984, p. 19; "The Supplement Story," pp. 12–13; Gentry, "MDs Rethinking Vitamins"; Cowley, "Vitamin Revolution."

45. "Suddenly, Vitamins Are Exciting Again," *Business Week,* 12 Feb. 1955, pp. 174–176, 178, 180.

46. "Taking Vitamins," p. 564.

# Index

Brand names are given in small capitals; page references in italics refer to illustrations.

Abbott Laboratories, 10, 30, 46, 131, 133

A-B-D-G VITAMIN CAPSULES (Kroger), 56, 57

Abzug, Bella, 159

acne, 110, 116, 219n1

ACNOTABS (Pannett), 86, 88, 109–124, 130; ingredients, 220n12

Action for Children's Television, 108

additives, 151, 152, 179. *See also* enrichment

ADEX TABLETS-10 D (Squibb), 26–27, *28*

advertising, 6, 14–31, 182; for ACNOTABS, 110–111; for ADEX TABLETS-10D, *28*; for BOTTLED SUNSHINE, 39; for cod-liver oil, 20, *21*, 22, *23*; directly to consumers, by proprietary firms, 86; for HYGEIA vegetables, *43*; for KITCHEN CRAFT WATERLESS COOKER, *15*; for ONE-A-DAY line, 89, 91, 92–95, *96*, 96–98, 99–100, 218n40; for OSCODAL, *24*; to pharmacists, by pharmaceutical industry, 65, 67–68, 86; radio, 92–93, 97–98; for RED HEART dog

biscuits, *16*; as reflection of desired reality, 203–204n19; science in, 102–103, 217n20; targeting children, 107–108, 180–182; television, 73, 98, 107–108; for VIGRAN, 73; for vitamin D, 50; for VITAMINS PLUS, 205n44; for Wisconsin Alumni Research Foundation, 45. *See also* marketing

Aikin, Mrs. Lee, 164

alar, 179

alcohol, 147, 150; and nutrition, 5, 182

alcoholism, 5, 129

"Alfred Hitchcock Hour," 73

ALKA-SELTZER (Miles), 86, 88–89, 92

*Alternative Medicine: A Guide* removed from Ellis Island immigration museum, 228n33

Alvarez, Walter C., 231n21

American Association of Retired Persons (AARP), 142, 143, 160

American Medical Association (AMA), 8, 9, 79, 103, 129, 185; Council on Foods and Nutrition, 134; denounces vitamin therapy, 77; department of nutrition, 82; on

AMA (*continued*)
  food processing, 136; Fraud Collection, 201n27; supports FDA, 162; and vitamin C, 81. *See also Journal of the American Medical Association*
American Pharmaceutical Association, 58–59
Anderson, Terence W., 82, 83
Anheuser Busch, 47
anti-oxidants, 186–187
anxieties, and vitamin marketing, 87. *See also* fear; guilt
"Are We Taking Too Many Vitamins?" (Brecher and Brecher), 128–129
ascorbic acid, *see* vitamin C
asthma, 129
atherosclerosis, 148
authority: FDA, over vitamins (*see* Food and Drug Administration); government, limits of, 126, 166; of pharmacists, 54, 55; of physicians, 54, 55; of science, 3, 12, 83, 85, 123, 180, 199n1
availability, restricted, of product, 154–155
avitaminosis, 2, 6, 29. *See also* vitamins: gross deficiencies in; *individual deficiency disorders*

Babcock, Stephen, 35
Babcock tester, 38
Baer, Rudolf, 116, 118, 119
balanced diet, 4, 182–183
Bass, Milton, 166, 170
beer, enriched, 50
Bell, Joseph, 215n69
beriberi, 2, 4, 5, 10, 85, 147
beta-carotene, 186–187
Better Business Bureau, National, 111
bile salts, 220n12
Biscuit and Cracker Manufacturers' Association, 49
Blackout Day, health food stores', 174, 229n48
Blatnik, John A., 163

Boards of Pharmacy, state: California, 69–70; Indiana, 56, 61; New York, 62, 63
BOND BREAD, 14
booklet and pamphlet distribution, 87, 95, 96–97, 100–101
Bosso, Angelo, 70
Bottled Beverages, Inc., 47
BOTTLED SUNSHINE (UltraVol Co.), 38, *39*
Boxer, Barbara, 175
Brecher, Ruth and Edward, 128–129
British Medical Association, 81
British Pharmacopeia, 16
Brown, Edmund G., 70
Brume, T. J., 38
BUGS BUNNY CHILDREN'S VITAMINS, 107
Bundesen, Herman N., *39*, 77
Buring, Julie, 187
butter-fat content, 35
B vitamins, 4, 5, 8–9, 25, 30, 192; and alcoholism, 5; $B_1$, 9, 10, 62, 131, 183; $B_2$, 62, 131, 183; $B_6$, 131, 183; $B_{12}$, 131
Byrd Antarctic Expedition, 25, 29

California Board of Pharmacy, 69–70
California Pharmaceutical Association, 69
cancer, 129, 147, 148, 157; and beta-carotene, 186–187; and vitamin C, 222n36
candy, fortified, 14
cavities (dental caries), 44
Center for Science in the Public Interest, 185
Centers for Disease Control, 176
cereals: advertising for, 20; enriched, 7, 44
chain stores, sales of vitamins by, 55
*Changing Times*, skeptical about vitamin C, 82
*Chemical Feast, The* (Turner), 137, 143; reviews of, 137–138

Chemix Corporation, 114, 115

*Chicago Tribune*, on benefits of vitamins, 185

children: fears for, exploited in advertising, 20–24 (*see also* "scientific motherhood"); as target market, 107, 181–182

CHOCKS multiple vitamins, 107

CHOCOLATE VIVATOSE, 14

choice: as freedom, 140, 145, 155; informed, 142, 143, 145, 156, 173

Chow, Bacon F., 223n23

cigarettes, 147, 150

Citizens for Health, 229n48

Clark, Paul, 65

cleanliness, appeals to, 26

clinical trials, 113, 115, 118, 121–122

Clissold, Jack W., 89, 90

cod-liver oil, 7, 8, 9, 14, 16–18, 25–26, 27, 32, 45–46, 75–76, 209n33; advertising for, 20, *21*, 22, *23*

Cohen, Jerome, 185–186

Committee on Recommended Dietary Allowances, 168

common cold, 75–84, 129. *See also* Pauling, Linus

Compton, Walter Amos, 88, 89, 103, 104–105, 106

conflict of interest, in science, 167–168

Congress, 145, 158–176; Delaney hearings (1950s), 151; House Hosmer bill hearings, 158–164; letters to, from consumers, 161, 164, 165, 171, 177, 191, 195; Proxmire Amendment hearings, 164–172. *See also individual bills and hearings*

consumer protection, 180; by FDA, 159, 161; as FDA rationale, 154–155; and patenting, 50

*Consumer Reports*, 188–191, 231n21

consumers: and choice, 140, 142, 143, 145; letters to Congress from, 171; letters to FDA from, 130, 145–157;

motivational studies of, 191–196; rights of, and Congress, 158, 163

*Consumers' Research Bulletin*, skepticism about vitamins, 98

Consumers Union, 188, 191, 231n21

Continental Machines, vitamin supplements at, 9–10

cooking, home, and vitamins, 4, 7

cornmeal and grits, enriched, 7

COSRAY, 40

costs: resulting from FDA regulations, 162; of vitamin production, 9

Council on Foods and Nutrition, American Medical Association, 134

CREAM OF WHEAT, 20

crepe label, 106–107, 131, 132–134, 137, 139, 223n12

dairy industry, 35, 36–37, 48. *See also* milk

Daniels, Amy L., 33

D'Argente, Russell, 114, 115

Davis, Adelle, 155

Davis, Marguerite, 17

De Kruif, Paul, 183

Delaney hearings, 151

department stores, vitamin sales by, 73, 205n42

Desmond, Ruth, 162

diet, average American: nutritional value of, 4, 8, 91–92, 128, 129, 148–149, 150, 165, 168, 180, 184, 187, 200n15; USDA survey of (1968), 135–136

Dilling, Kirkpatrick, 134

discount drugstores, 73

displays, window and counter, pharmacists', *64*, 64–65, *66*, 72

door-to-door sales of vitamins, 74

double-blind testing, 114, 115, 117, 118

Douglas, Paul H., 166

druggists, *see* pharmacists

drug manufacturers, *see* pharmaceutical industry

*Drug Topics*, 55, 56; on the common cold, 76; on market shares, 213n26; on ONE-A-DAY advertising, 218n40; window displays in, *64, 66, 72*

Eddy, Walter H., 9
educational promotions, 105
Edwards, Douglas, 73
efficacy, therapeutic, 113, 120–122, 141, 149
ELDERTONIC VITAMIN-MINERAL SUPPLEMENT, 31
Eli Lilly and Company, 46, 100, 122
Ellis Island immigration museum, 228n33
empirical evidence, 118, 124
enrichment of foodstuffs and cosmetics, 7, 14, 36, 40, 67, 151; recommended by AMA and NAS, 136; through irradiation (*see* irradiation)
ergesterol, irradiated, 46, 47
ethylene dichloride, 209n33
E.T.—THE EXTRA-TERRESTRIAL CHILDREN'S CHEWABLE VITAMINS, 31
evidence: conflicting, 166; consumers' interpretation of, 157; empirical, 118, 124; of harm, 152, 159, 227n13; inconclusive, in science, 11–12, 139, 143, 144

FDA, *see* Food and Drug Administration
fear, arousal of, in advertising, 19, 20–22
Federal Trade Commission (FTC), 30, 88, 89, 98, 103, 108, 111, 201n27, 216n5
Federation of Homemakers, 162
Fleischmann's (yeast manufacturer), 47
FLINTSTONES children's vitamins, 107–108
flour and bread, enriched, 7, 14, 67, 151
fluoride, 179

folic acid, 131, 176
Food and Drug Act of 1906, 172; McNary-Maples Amendment to (1930), 223n12
Food and Drug Administration (FDA), 11; and ACNOTABS, 111–114, 120; backs down on 1962 regulatory proposals, 130–131; and *The Chemical Feast*, 137–138; and classification of vitamins, 58–59; commissions *A Study of Health Practices and Opinions*, 193, 194, 232n38; in congressional hearings, 145 (*see also individual bills and hearings*); and consumer protection, 154–155; credibility of, 125; denounces vitamin therapy, 77; GRAS list, 138, 151; and harmful substances (*see* harm, evidence of); and the Hosmer bill, 158–159; and labeling, 216n5 (*see also* labeling and packaging); letters to, from consumers, 130, 145–157, 191, 195; and Miles ONE-A-DAY line, 88, 89–92; and the Nutritional Labeling and Education Act of 1990, 174; premarketing conferences with manufacturers, 88, 216n15; and the Proxmire Amendment, 164–172, 173; and RDAs, 78, 224n33 (*see also* recommended dietary allowances); regulatory proposals and rebuffs, 106–107, 127–128, 130, 131–136, 222n8; replies to consumer mail, 153–154; skeptical of vitamins, 183; and vitamin C, 81, 138–139, 141; vitamin research by, 112; and VITAMINS PLUS, 29–30
Food and Nutrition Board, National Research Council, 106, 133, 134, 162, 224n33
Food, Drug and Cosmetics Act of 1938, 59, 113; amendments to, 121, 122–123, 125, 141
food faddism, 149. *See also* quackery

food processing, and nutrient loss, 4, 6, 128, 136, 151, 180, 191–192
fraud, 77, 160, 169, 177, 180; and the rhetoric of science, 91. *See also* consumer protection; quackery
Fraud Collection, AMA, 201n27
freedom-of-choice argument, 140, 145, 155
Friendly, Henry J., 170
fruit, 7, 182; and the common cold, 81
Fuller Brush Company, 74
Funk, Casimir, 13

*Gang's All Here, The* (film), 10
General Foods, 168
"generally recognized as safe" (GRAS) list, FDA, 138, 151
General Mills, 25
Gershoff, Stanley N., 137
Gilmour, Gene, 64
*Glamour:* on benefits of vitamins, 185; reports beta-carotene study, 186
Glover, A. J., 37
Goddard, James Lee, 132, 133, 139, 147
Goodall's Laboratories, 38
*Good Housekeeping:* advertising in, 18, *21, 23,* 92, 205n44; endorses vitamin use, 93; explodes vitamin "myths," 128–129; and FLINT-STONES vitamin controversy, 107; letters to, about vitamins, 14; motivational survey by, 192–193; and vitamins for skin, 9
Good Housekeeping Bureau, 9, 18
gout, 16
Great Depression, 6–7, 25, 30
*Great Vitamin Hoax, The* (Tatkon), 169–170
"Great Vitamin Scare, The" (*New Republic* article), 98–99
Green (chain stores), vitamin sales by, 55
grocers, vitamin sales by, 55–59, 73,

205n42; market share, 68–69; and state Boards of Pharmacy, 56, 61, 69–70
GROVE'S VITAMINS, 67
guilt, arousal of, in advertising, 19, 20, 25, 26–27
György, Paul, 223n23

harm, evidence of, 152, 159, 227n13
Harper, Alfred E., 168
*Harper's Bazaar,* VITAMINS PLUS advertised in, 205n44
Harris, David H., 137
Harrison, Harold E., 223n23
Harrow, Benjamin, 63
Hart, E. B., 34, 37
Hatch, K. L., 37–38
Hatch, Orrin G., 175–176
Hatch-Richardson bill (Health Freedom Act), 176, 177
heads, bodyless, patent life-support system for, 211n54
Health Action Committee, 160, 164
health food stores' Blackout Day, 174, 229n48
Health Freedom Act (Hatch-Richardson bill), 176, 177
Health Professions Assistance Act, 171–172
Health Research Group, 142–143, 171–172
Herbert, Victor, 169, 228n33
HEW, *see* U.S. Department of Health, Education, and Welfare
*Hoard's Dairyman,* 37
Hoffman, Nicholas von, 159
Hoffmann-La Roche Company, 193
Holstein, Lisa W., 225n47
home cooking, and vitamins, 4, 7
homeopathic pharmacopeia, 62
hope, 93; arousal of, in advertising, 19, 20, 22, 25, 32
hormones, bovine growth, 179
Hoskins, William, 42
Hosmer, Craig, 158, 159, 164

housewife survey (Miles Laboratories), 192–193
H.R. 643 (Hosmer bill), 158–159, 160
Hughes, Cheryl, 229n48
Hutt, Peter Barton, 159
*Hygeia* (magazine), 9; advertising in, *15*, 18, *24*, 25, *43*; letters published in, 14
Hygeia Nursing Bottle Company, *43*
HYGEIA vegetables, *43*

"ignorance claims," 225n47
Ihde, Aaron, 207n3
Independent Grocers' Alliance (IGA), vitamin sales by, *56*
Indiana Board of Pharmacy, 56, 61
Indiana Supreme Court, and the Kroger case, 61
informed choice, 142, 143, 156, 173
insulin, patenting of, 36
International Vitamin Corporation, 67, 209n33
irradiation, ultraviolet, patenting of, 34, 35–53, 206n2

*JAMA, see Journal of the American Medical Association*
Jewels Pharmaceuticals, 112
Johnson, Ogden C., 160
Jolliffe, Norman Hayhurst, 5
Jolly, Charles N., 161
*Journal of Biological Chemistry*, 33
*Journal of Nutrition Education*, 105
*Journal of the American Medical Association*, 97; skeptical about vitamin C, 82
juice, 182

Kauffmann Pharmacy (Hatboro, Pa.), *76*
"Keep 'em coming!" (*Drug Topics* cartoon), *60*
Kefauver-Harris Amendment (1966) to Food, Drug and Cosmetics Act of 1938, 121, 122–123, 125

Kelly, Patrick, 211n54
Kelsey, Francis, 122
Kelter, Joseph J., 115–116, 118, 119, 123
Kennedy, Edward M., 164
Kessler, David, 174
King, Charles Glen, 81
KITCHEN CRAFT WATERLESS COOKER, 14, *15*
Kresge (chain store), vitamin sales by, 55
Kroger Grocery and Baking Company, 55–59; litigation, 57–59, 61

labeling and packaging, vitamin, 88, 89–92, 123; of ACNOTABS, 111, 112, 114; consumer's view of, 150; crepe label, 106–107, 131, 132–134, 137, 139, 223n12; FDA jurisdiction over, 216n5; under H.R. 643, 159; of "intrinsically injurious" products, 159; orthodox science and, 87, 120; proposed FDA regulations of 1940, 127–128; proposed FDA regulations of 1962, 131; proposed FDA regulations of 1973, 140–143; state Board of Pharmacy classification, 61
lactic acid, 30
*Ladies' Home Journal*, on benefits of vitamins, 8–9, 185
laetrile, 157
Larrick, George, 90, 91, 130
Lederle Laboratories, 100
legislation: science defined by, 121, 122–123, 125; scientific expertise and, 123. *See also individual bills and amendments*
letters: to Congress, from consumers, 161, 164, 165, 171, 177, 191, 195; to *Consumer Reports*, 189–191; to the FDA, 130–131; to the FDA, from consumers, 130, 145–157, 191, 195; to the FDA, from physicians and researchers, 223n23; to *Good House-*

*keeping,* from consumers, 14; in *Hygeia,* 14

Lever Brothers, 86, 99

Ley, Herbert, 134, 135

*Life* magazine, ONE-A-DAY advertising in, 102–103

lifesupport machine, patent, for bodyless heads, 211n54

liquor, *see* alcohol

litigation, 158; ACNOTABS, 114; blocking FDA regulations, 170; about vitamins as drugs vs. food, 57–59, 61

"Lum 'n' Abner" radio show, 93

LYSOL, 26

*McCall's,* on vitamins and diet, 182, 185

McCarthy, John, 116, 118

McCollum, Elmer V., 17, 35

MCKESSON'S HIGH POTENCY COD LIVER OIL (McKesson and Robbins), 22

MacNamara, Patrick V., 104

McNary-Maples Amendment (1930) to Food and Drug Act of 1906, 223n12

*Mademoiselle,* 79

mail, *see* letters

mail order vitamin sales, 73

margarine, enrichment of, 7, 36–37

Marion County Superior Court, Indiana, 61

market fragmentation, 31

marketing: to children, 107–108, 181–182; and educational campaigns, 101, 102–103; window and counter displays, pharmacists', *64,* 64–65, *66, 72*; to women, 31. *See also* advertising

Marks, Harry Milton, 220n18

Maryland, University of, vitamin C study, 82

Mayer, Gerald F., 153

Mayo Clinic, 10

MDR, *see* minimum daily requirement

Mead Johnson Company, 46, 100, 135

*Medicine Show, The* (Consumers Union), 231n21

megadosing, 81, 141, 149, 160

MEGA-MEN, 31

Mellanby, Edward, 17

Merck & Company, 100, 133

Merrill, William S., Pharmaceutical Company, 122

Metz, H. A., Laboratories, 22

Miles Laboratories, 86–108, 109, 124, 133, 142, 160, 161, 191; fights crepe label, 132–133; motivational surveys by, 191–193; premarketing conferences with FDA, 88–92, 216n15

milk, 7; and B vitamins, 6; fortified, 48. *See also* dairy industry

Miller, Clinton, 166

Miner, Carl, 42

minimum daily requirement (MDR), 127, 131

Minnesota, University of, common cold study at, 77, 79

"Mr. Ed" TV show, 73

moderation, based on science, 104

*Modern Brewer,* 50

Morrison, F. B., 37, 38, 47

Morrison, William, 114, 115

Mory, A.V.H., 49

motherhood, "scientific," 19–20, 27, 93, 202n2, 204n21, 217n20

motivational surveys of vitamin users, 191–196

multivitamin supplements, 131, 133

Nader, Ralph, 138, 142–143

*Nason's Cod Liver Oil,* 25

*Nation, The,* on Pauling and vitamin C, 79

National Academy of Sciences, 133, 168, 173; on food processing, 136. *See also* National Research Council

● ● ● ● ● ● ● ● ● ● ● ● ● ● ● ● ● ● ● ● ● ● ● ● ● ● ● ● ● ● ● ● ● ● ● ●

National Association of Food Supplement Manufacturers, 134

National Association of Retail Druggists, 58–59

"National Barndance" radio show, 92

National Better Business Bureau, 111

National Congress on Medical Quackery (1961), 130

National Health Alliance, 229n48

National Health Federation, 130–131, 141–142, 145, 158, 160, 166

National Heart and Lung Institutes Bill, Proxmire Amendment attached to, 172

National Institutes of Health, 82, 122

National Nutritional Foods Association, 160, 170, 229n48

National Oil Products Company, 48

National Research Council, 138, 167–168, 189; Food and Nutrition Board, 106, 133, 134, 162; and vitamin C, 81

National Retired Teachers Association, 142, 143, 160

National Vitamin Foundation, 100–101

"negative appeal" advertising, 19, 29. *See also* guilt

Nelson, E. M., 89, 90, 91

Newberry (chain store), vitamin sales by, 55

*New Republic*, skepticism about vitamins, 98–99

*Newsweek*: on benefits of vitamins, 185; on Pauling and vitamin C, 79; reports beta-carotene study, 186

New York Board of Pharmacy, 62, 63

New York Department of Consumer Affairs, 107

*New Yorker, The*, vitamin cartoon in, 30

New York State Food Merchants' Association, 62–63

*New York Times*: on benefits of vitamins, 63, 185; reports beta-carotene

study, 186; skeptical about vitamin C, 82

niacin (nicotinic acid), 131, 200n7

Northern California Retail Druggists' Association, 69

nutrition, 6–7; and workforce productivity, 9. *See also* balanced diet; diet, average American

*Nutrition Action* (Center for Science in the Public Interest), 185

Nutritional Labeling and Education Act, 174

oatmeal, 44

Office of Legislative Services, FDA, 153

oleomargarine, enriched, 7, 36–37; licensing of, 47, 52; research into, 42

One-A-Day line (Miles), 86–88, 109, 124, 161, 169; B-complex, 95; critics of, 98–99; A & D, 87, 89–94, *94*, 95; motivational research for, 191–192; Multiple Vitamin Tablets, 96; Plus Iron, 101–102, 217n36

*Operation Petticoat* (film), 183–184

*Organic Gardening and Farming*, 136

"orthomolecular medicine," Pauling's, 78

Oscodal, 22

Ovaltine, 14

Owen, George M., 223n23

pancreatin, 220n12

Pannett Company, 86, 109–124

pantothenic acid, 131

*Parents' Magazine*, advertising in, 18, *28*, *45*, 92, 93–94, *94*

Parke-Davis, 46, 86

"Password," TV quiz show, 73

pasta, enriched, 7

patents: administered by university research departments, 42–53, 208n25; Steenbock process, 34, 35–42, 208–209n29, 209n33 paternalism, FDA appearance of, 145, 156, 168

Pauling, Linus, 54, 74–75, 78–84, 123, 138, 163, 214n41, 222n36

Pearson, W. N., 223n23

pellagra, 2, 200n7

pepsin, 220n12

petitions, to the FDA, 146

pets, vitamin supplements for, 14, 16, *16*

Pfizer & Company, 30, 133

pharmaceutical industry, 8, 85–86, 139; on clinical testing, 122; marketing to pharmacists, 65, 67–68; marketing to public, 19–31; and nonpharmacist vitamin sales, 58–59; and the Steenbock irradiation patent, 47, 52; vitamins as percentage of sales, 30–31

Pharmaceutical Manufacturers Association, 133, 224n36

pharmacists: authority of, 54, 55; distribute ONE-A-DAY booklets, 95; limited by medical profession, 205n42; oppose grocers' vitamin sales, 55, 56–59; professionalism of, 59–61, *60*, 64–65, 67–68, *70*, 70–73, 74, 84; vitamin marketing by, 181–182

phocomelia, 122

phone calls, to Congress, 177. *See also* letters: to Congress

physicians: authority of, 54, 55; consumer skepticism about, 83, 126, 153; lack of consensus among, 139, 185–186; professionalism of, 64, 84, 85; review Miles advertising, 89; uneasy about placebos, 116

Pineapple Producers Cooperative, 25

placebos, 115, 116

polyneuritis, 5, 13

POLY-VI-SOL, 31

Postum Cereal Company, 49

press, popular, and vitamin lore, 3–12. *See also individual publications*

print promotions, 92, 93–94; for ACNOTABS, 110; Squibb's, 73

productivity, workforce, and nutrition, 9

professionalism, 59–61, 85; of pharmacists, 64–65, 67–68, *70*, 70–73, 74, 84, 85; of physicians, 64, 83, 84, 85. *See also* authority

Prohibition (Volstead Act), 142

Proxmire, William, 165–166, 167–168, 169, 171–172, 175

Proxmire Amendment, 126, 158, 164–170 (*see also* Vitamin Amendment of 1976); passes, 171–172; Senate hearings on, 164–170

Public Health Service, U.S., 82

quackery, 11, 103, 104–105, 123, 129–130, 169, 177, 228n33. *See also* consumer protection; fraud

QUAKER OATS, 44, 46, 52

"Queen for a Day" radio show, 93

"Quiz Kids, The," radio show, 92

radio promotions, 92–93, 97–98

radon, 179

rationing, World War II, 10, 67

*Reader's Digest*, 129

Reasoner, Harry, 73

"reason why" advertising, 19

recommended dietary allowances (RDAs), 78, 131, 140, 141, 148, 161–162, 167–168, 170, 171, 172, 173–174, 188

RED HEART DOG BISCUITS, 14, 16, *16*

respectability, scientific and medical, and the ONE-A-DAY line, 103–108. *See also* professionalism

Reynolds, J. A., 76

rheumatism, 16

Richards, Evelleen, 221–222n36

Richardson, Bill, 175

rickets, 4, 16, 22, *39*, 44, 85, 147; in advertising, *24*
Robinson, Miles, 166
Rodale, J. I., 136
Roy, William R., 161
Russell, Harry L., 35, 40, 42, 47, 51, 208–209n29

"Sally Forth" (cartoon), 184
*Saturday Evening Post*: advertising in, 25; on vitamin C, 83
scarlet fever, 27
Schaefer, Arnold, 134
Schmidt, Alexander, 140, 144, 148, 159, 166, 168, 169, 170–171
science: in advertising, 18, 25, 87, 102–103, 217n20; authority of, 3, 12, 83, 85, 123, 180, 199n1; compromised by conflict of interest, 167–168; conflicting definitions of, 80–81, 117–118, 124, 126–127, 144, 180–181, 196, 197; contradictory evidence and conclusions in, 11–12, 139, 143, 144, 166, 176, 196, 224n33; defined by legislation, 123, 125; evolving, 152, 158; and "ignorance claims," 225n47; mainstream vs. quackish, 109; orthodox, at the FDA, 120, 147–148, 155, 156, 159, 160–161, 169–170, 176–177; at public institutions, 207n12 (*see also* Wisconsin Alumni Research Foundation); in retreat from the public domain, 202n37; rhetoric of, 91, 110, 124, 179; and testing procedures, 113–117, 118
*Science* (magazine), 34; reviews *The Chemical Feast*, 137–138; skepticism about vitamins, 103
*Science Digest*, 129
"scientific motherhood," 19–20, 27, 93, 202n2, 204n21, 217n20
scurvy, 2, 4, 13
Sebrell, William, 138

self-help movement, 74
self-medication, 83
Senate Select Committee on Nutrition and Human Needs, 106
Senate Special Committee on Aging, 104–105
Sereda, Joseph P., 38, 40
Shane, Theodore, 114, 115
Shuman, Howard E., 165, 166, 172, 227n19
single grain ration experiment, Steenbock's, 35
skin, vitamins applied to, 9, 14
Slichter, Charles, 42
Smith, Sybil L., 9
soap, enriched, 9, 14, 40, 201n27
sodium nitrate, 151
soil depletion, 128
Speckart, Herbert R., 64–65
Squibb, E. R., 46, 86, 99; advertising by, 20, *21*, 22, *23*, 25, 26
SQUIBB ADEX TABLETS-10 D, 26–27, *28*
STAMMS (Standard Brands), 99
Stare, Frederick J., 79, 80, 84, 134, 215n69
Starr, Paul, 199n1
Steenbock, Harry, 7, 33–53, 54, 168, 206–207n3
stimulants, 150
Stocking, S. Holly, 225n47
Stone, Irwin, 78
"Stop that cold!" (window display), *76*
STRESSTAB HIGH-POTENCY STRESS FORMULA VITAMINS, 31
STUART PRE-NATAL TABLETS, 31
*Study of Health Practices and Opinions, A* (National Analysts, Inc.), 193, 194, 232n21
Supermarket Institute, 62
Swann, John, 221n29

Tatkon, M. Daniel, 169–170
teeth, and vitamins, 44

television advertising, 73, 98, 107
testimonials in advertising, 25, 29
thalidomide, 122
therapeutic efficacy, 113, 120–122, 141, 149
thiamine (vitamin $B_1$), 9, 10, 62, 131
Thompson, J. Walter, advertising agency, 20, 25
*Time* magazine, on benefits of vitamins, 184–185
tobacco, 147, 150; and nutrition, 182
*Today's Health*, 77
toothpaste advertising, 19
Toronto, University of, vitamin C study, 81–82
toxicity of vitamins, 227n13
Tracy, Dr. (ACNOTABS chemist), 114
Turner, James S., 137, 143

"Ubiquitous Vitamin Preparations, The" (*Consumers' Research Bulletin* article), 98
ultraviolet light, irradiation with, *see* irradiation
UltraVol Company, 38
*Uncle Sam—Last of the Big Time Spenders* (Proxmire), 165
U.S. Court of Appeals, 170
U.S. Department of Agriculture (USDA): advises B vitamins for nursing mothers, 9; on American diet, 103; on fruit and the common cold, 81; nutritional survey by, 150; supports vitamin enrichment of foodstuffs, 7; surveys American diet (1968), 135–136
U.S. Department of Health, Education, and Welfare (HEW), 134, 148, 152; FDA (*see* Food and Drug Administration)
U.S. Department of Health and Human Services, 176, 189

*U.S. News & World Report*, skeptical about vitamin C, 82
United States Pharmacopeia (USP), 62, 63
U.S. Vitamin and Pharmaceutical Corporation, 100
University of Maryland vitamin C study, 82
University of Minnesota vitamin C study, 77, 79
University of Toronto vitamin C study, 81–82
Upjohn Company, 99, 133, 209–210n33
UVO (Wisconsin Alumni Research Foundation), 48, 52

vegetables, 182
vegetarianism, 182
VICTORY vitamins (Abbott), 10
VIGRAN (Squibb), 73
VIMMS (Lever Brothers), 99
VIOSTEROL, 46
vitamin A, 25, 26, 30, 36, 58, 62, 131, 183, 220n12, 227n13; and acne, 114, 117, 118; in advertising, *21, 22, 23*; applied to skin, 9; and beta-carotene, 186; discovery of, 4; product labeling claims for, 90–91; RDA disputed, 173; Steenbock's irradiation process, 42, 206n2; and vision, 4, 17, 177
Vitamin Amendment of 1976, 172, 173. *See also* Proxmire Amendment
vitamin B, *see* B vitamins
vitamin C, 25, 62, 131, 138, 171, 220n12, 227n13; and the common cold, 2, 75–84, 177; and the FDA, 138–139, 141, 148–149; and Linus Pauling, 54, 74–75, 78–84, 214n41, 222n36; RDA disputed, 173; and scurvy, 4
*Vitamin C and the Common Cold* (Pauling), 79

vitamin D, 25, 26, 36, 62, 131, 151, 209n33, 227n13; in advertising, 22, *24, 43*; applied to skin, 9, 14; product labeling claims for, 91; and rickets, 4, 16; in soap, 40; Steenbock's irradiation patent, 34, 35–53
vitamin E, 131, 149, 185–186; and heart ailments, 2
Vitamin Information Bureau, 100
"Vitamin Month" marketing drive, New Jersey, 65, *66*
Vitamin Nutrition Information Service, Hoffmann-La Roche Company, 193
*Vitamin Power* (Aero and Rick), 184
vitamins, 1; consumer profile studies, 191–196; cost of production of, 9; discovery and popularizing of, 2–12; as drugs vs. food, 57–59, 61–62, 140; FDA regulation of (*see* Food and Drug Administration); gross deficiencies in, 2, 14, 85, 179 (*see also individual disorders*); litigation about, 57–59, 61; marketing of, 55–77, *64*, 64–65, *66*, *71*; market shares, 213n26; nonpharmacist sales of, 68–69, 73–74; percentage of Americans using, 194; prescribed by physicians, 201n24; sales figures, 11; subclinical deficiencies in, 97, 128–129; toxicity of, 227n13. *See also individual vitamins*
"Vitamins and Your Health" (National Vitamin Foundation), 100–101
"Vitamins, Minerals and Americans," pamphlet, 105
VITAMINS PLUS, 29–30, 182, 205n42, 205n44
VITA-RAY CREAM, 14
VITEX (National Oil Products Co.), 48
VITROETTS, 6
Volstead Act (Prohibition), 142
V. V. VITAWATER, 5

Wade, Jeff, 101
Wade Advertising Agency, 99, 101
Wadsworth, Ruth, 4
Waldorf Astoria Hotel, 30
Wallace, Robert, 108
WARF, *see* Wisconsin Alumni Research Foundation
*Washington Post* breaks thalidomide story, 122
"What do Dietary Supplements and Dinosaurs Have in Common?" (poster), 174, *175*
Wheelock, C. E., jam makers, 47
Whelan drugstore, Philadelphia, *63*
White, Philip, 82
White, Suzanne, 219n2, 222n8
WHITES' COD LIVER OIL CONCENTRATE, 26
Wilder, Russell, 10
Wiles, Russell, 42
Wilkie, Leighton, 9–10
Williams, Roger J., 161–162
window and counter displays: health food stores' Blackout Day (1993), 174; pharmacists', *64*, 64–65, *66*, *71*
Winthrop Chemical Company, 46
Wisconsin Alumni Research Foundation, 7, 34, 42–53, 208–209n29, 210n48, 211n53
WITHIN ADVANCED MULTIVITAMIN FOR WOMEN, 31
women, 14, 129, 192–193; marketing to, 31, as mothers, 17–27. *See also* children; *Good Housekeeping*; motherhood; *Parents' Magazine*
Woodruff, Calvin, 135
Woolworth (chain store), vitamin sales by, 55
workforce productivity, 9–10
World War II, 181; and industrial productivity, 9–10; military's use of vitamins during, 127, 181; rationing during, and nutrition, 10, 67

Wyatt, Wendell, 163

Wyeth Laboratories, 133

*Yearbook of Dermatology*, 116

*You Can Do It! Senator Proxmire's Exer-*

*cise, Diet and Relaxation Plan* (Proxmire), 165

"You have the upper hand" (*Drug
Topics* cartoon), *71*

Young, James Harvey, 172

## About the Author

Rima D. Apple teaches at the University of Wisconsin–Madison, where she holds a joint appointment in the Department of Consumer Science and the Women's Studies Program. The author of *Mothers and Medicine: A Social History of Infant Feeding, 1890–1950* (1987) and editor of *Women, Health and Medicine in America: A Historical Handbook* (1990, 1992), she has lectured extensively both here and abroad on the history of science, history of medicine, and women's history.